American Catholic Hospitals

Critical Issues in Health and Medicine

Edited by Rima D. Apple, University of Wisconsin–Madison,
and Janet Golden, Rutgers University, Camden

Growing criticism of the U.S. health care system is coming from consumers, politicians, the media, activists, and health care professionals. Critical Issues in Health and Medicine is a collection of books that explores these contemporary dilemmas from a variety of perspectives, among them political, legal, historical, sociological, and comparative, and with attention to crucial dimensions such as race, gender, ethnicity, sexuality, and culture.

For a list of titles in the series, see the last page of the book.

American Catholic Hospitals

A Century of Changing Markets and Missions

Barbra Mann Wall

Rutgers University Press

New Brunswick, New Jersey, and London

First paperback edition, 2016

Library of Congress Cataloging–in–Publication Data

Wall, Barbra Mann.
 American Catholic hospitals : a century of changing markets and missions / Barbra Mann Wall.
  p. cm. — (Critical issues in health and medicine)
  Includes bibliographical references and index.
  ISBN 978-0-8135-4940-8 (hardcover : alk. paper)—ISBN 978-0-8135-7644-2 (pbk. : alk. paper)
  1. Catholic hospitals—United States—History—20th century. 2. Catholic hospitals—United States—History—21st century. 3. Social change—United States—History—20th century. 4. Social change—United States—History—21st century. 5. Catholic hospitals—United States—Marketing—History. 6. Catholic hospitals—Social aspects—United States—History. 7. Nuns—United States—History. 8. Nursing—United States—Religious aspects—History. 9. Medical care—United States—Religious aspects—Catholic Church—History. I. Title.

 RA975.C37W33 2011
 362.11008'2—dc22   2010017322

A British Cataloging-in-Publication record for this book is available from the British Library.

Visit our website: http://rutgerspress.rutgers.edu

Manufactured in the United States of America

For my parents, Billy and Jean Mann

Contents

Illustrations and Tables

Illustrations

Tables

Acknowledgments

I am indebted to the staffs of several archives for their assistance: Donna Dahl, archivist, Alexian Brothers Provincial Archives, Arlington Heights, Illinois; Carole Prietto, archivist, Daughters of Charity National Health System, St. Louis, Missouri; Kathleen Washy, archivist, University of Pittsburgh Medical Center/Mercy Hospital Archives, Pittsburgh, Pennsylvania; Loretta Greene, archivist, and Peter F. Schmid, CA, visual resources archivist, Providence Archives, Mother Joseph Province, Seattle, Washington; Kathy Urbanic, archivist, Sisters of Saint Joseph of Rochester Archives, Rochester, New York; Timothy Oh, archivist, Mercy Hospital and Medical Center, Chicago, Illinois; Sister Joella Cunnane, RSM, archivist, Sisters of Mercy, Chicago, Illinois; Susan Eason, archivist, and Eric J. Hartmann, assistant archivist, Catholic Archives of Texas, Austin, Texas, and the staff at the Austin History Center; the Chicago Archdiocese Archives staff; and the Chicago Historical Museum staff. At Seton Family of Hospitals, Austin, Texas, I thank Carl R. McQueary, senior archivist and historian; Sister Helen Brewer, DC, chair, Seton Board of Trustees; and Sister Pat Elder, DC, ambassador for Dell Children's Medical Center.

I used a number of oral histories for the book. I offer a special acknowledgment to Sisters Barbara Lynaugh, SSJ, and Mary John van Atta, SSJ, from the Sisters of Saint Joseph of Rochester, New York, for helping me set up oral histories with the sisters who worked in Selma, Alabama. A special thanks goes to those sisters: Sisters Mary Paul Geck, SSJ; Barbara Lum, SSJ; Josepha Twomey, SSJ; and Catherine Teresa Martin, SSJ. I am also grateful to others who granted me interviews: Bernita McTernan, senior vice-president for governance, Mission Integration, and Philanthropy at Catholic Healthcare West; Sister Sheila Lyne, RSM, CEO, Mercy Hospital and Medical Center, Chicago, Illinois; Sister Felice Sauers, RSM; and Sister Helene Lentz, CSJ.

Funding for this Scholarly Works project was made possible by Grant 1G13 IM009691–01 from the National Library of Medicine, National Institutes of Health, Department of Health and Human Services. The views expressed in any written publication do not necessarily reflect the official policies of the Department of Health and Human Services nor does mention of trade names, commercial practices, or organizations imply endorsement by the U.S.

government. Funding also was provided by the University of Pennsylvania's University Research Foundation Grant, the Trustee Council of Penn Women Summer Fellowship Award, a Fichter Grant from the Association for the Sociology of Religion, and an H15 Grant for Historical Research by the American Association for the History of Nursing.

Portions of the following articles are used with permission of the publishers: "Conflict and Compromise: Catholic and Public Hospital Partnerships," *Nursing History Review* 18 (2010): 100–117, published by Springer Publishing Company; "Catholic Nursing Sisters and Brothers and Racial Justice in Mid-20th-Century America," *Advances in Nursing Science* 32, no. 2 (2009): E81; "Religion and Gender in a Men's Hospital and School of Nursing, 1866–1969," *Nursing Research* 58, no. 3 (2009): 158–165; and "Catholic Sister Nurses in Selma, Alabama, 1940–1972," *Advances in Nursing Science* 32, no. 1 (2009): 91–102. The last three articles were published by Wolters Klewer Publishers.

The book was shaped by the intellectually stimulating environment at the University of Pennsylvania. Joan Lynaugh and Karen Buhler-Wilkerson were superb mentors. Besides sharing their expertise, they were always encouraging and available, and it has been a pleasure to work with them. Unfortunately, Karen did not live to see the publication of this book, but my memories of her inspired my words, and her encouraging spirit comforted me during moments of stress and struggle. My colleagues at the Barbara Bates Center for the Study of the History of Nursing have given freely of their time, expertise, friendship, and support: Julie Fairman, Patricia O'Brien D'Antonio, Jean Whelan, Cynthia Connolly, Ellen Baer, and Julie Sochalski. Betsy Weiss provided valuable staff assistance. Linda Aiken and her colleagues in the Center for Health Outcomes and Policy Research offered insightful comments on chapter 5.

I am grateful to other colleagues: Arlene Keeling and Barbara Brodie from the University of Virginia, who continued to provide support and friendship; Susanne Malchau Dietz from Denmark, who presented at conferences with me and was a great traveling companion; Carmen Mangion, Carolyn Bowden, and other colleagues from the History of Women Religious in England and Ireland organization; Rima Apple, Janet Golden, Doreen Valentine, Marlie Wasserman, and Peter Mickulas, who read the manuscript and offered important suggestions; and the reviewers for Rutgers University Press.

My final comments are for family and friends. I acknowledge the love and support from my sister and best friend, Debra Mann. My son, Austin, continues to inspire and delight me. Cynthia Cantwell has provided friend-ship and encouragement to me for over forty years. And I could not have writ-ten this book without the help of my husband, Robyn, whose patience and love kept me going. He read the drafts and edited almost every word, and he bolstered my confidence at crucial times. Finally, I acknowledge the love and support, in so many ways, of my parents, Billy and Jean Mann, who would have been proud of me even if I had never written a book. It is to them that this book is dedicated.

Abbreviations

AHA	American Hospital Association
AHERF	Allegheny Health Education and Research Foundation
AMA	American Medical Association
ANA	American Nurses Association
BBA	Balanced Budget Act of 1997
CFA	Congregatio Fratrum Alexianorum (Congregation of Alexian Brothers)
CFFC	Catholics for a Free Choice
CHA	Catholic Health Association (originally the Catholic Hospital Association)
CHW	Catholic Healthcare West
CIC	Catholic Interracial Council
Columbia/HCA	Columbia/Hospital Corporation of America
CNA	California Nurses Association
CSJ	Congregation of Saint Joseph
DC	Daughters of Charity of Saint Vincent de Paul
DCNHS	Daughters of Charity National Health System
ESP	Economic Security Program
FSM	Franciscan Sisters of Mary
NCCB	National Conference of Catholic Bishops
OP	Dominicans (Order of Friars Preachers)
PMHS	Pittsburgh Mercy Health System
RSM	Religious Sisters of Mercy
SC	Sisters of Charity
SEIU	Service Employees International Union
SJ	Society of Jesus (Jesuits)
SP	Sisters of Providence
SSE	Society of Saint Edmund
SSJ	Sisters of Saint Joseph
SSM	Franciscan Sisters of Saint Mary
UPMC	University of Pittsburgh Medical Center
USCCB	U.S. Conference of Catholic Bishops
WSNA	Washington State Nurses Association

American Catholic Hospitals

Chapter 1

From Sisters in Habits to Men in Suits

The public face of Catholic authority has always been decidedly male; it is indeed ironic, then, that the overwhelming majority of Catholic hospitals in the United States were established and originally managed by women. While mission driven, these Catholic sisters, or nuns, were nevertheless skillful business managers who learned to understand fully and work within the often perilous hospital marketplace.[1] The exception to female-founded institutions was the hospital established by the Alexian Brothers from Aachen, Germany, who were founded to care for the sick and dying. Using U.S. Catholic women's religious congregations (sometimes called orders or communities) and one men's congregation as vehicles for examination, this book provides a historical analysis of the changing identity and influence of Catholic hospitals from the Great Depression to the present. Many of these changes are emblematic of how the health care system as a whole has changed. Indeed, much of the argument I make applies to the rest of the hospital sector: the effect of large changes in the economics of health care; the spread of health insurance and negotiations between the hospitals and insurers; the increase in government funding and regulation; authority issues; ideas about a good work atmosphere; and unions as a danger to hospitals. For Catholic hospitals, in particular, a gender disparity developed in leadership as institutions run primarily by religious women came to be administered, for the most part, by men.[2]

In the United States, religious-affiliated hospitals play a significant role in delivering health care to medically underserved, diverse, and poverty-stricken communities. The Catholic Church, in particular, is a major stakeholder in the health care field. Yet few historians have investigated the importance of religious-affiliated hospitals for U.S. society and the inevitable awkwardness when they attempt directly to shape medical policies in a diverse milieu. This is especially important in the health care arena, where life, birth, and death are critical benchmarks for quality and justification for services.

Catholic hospitals began as individual, stand-alone institutions, and they have a long and rich history in the United States. They were established with religious missions to care for both Catholics and non-Catholics. Sisters and brothers served with distinction despite considerable hardship. These hospitals experienced massive transformations, however, mainly in the last forty years as modern medicine made new demands and the number of Catholic women and men in religious orders plummeted. The dramatic evolution of Catholic hospitals must be seen within the context of landmark events such as the passage of Medicare and Medicaid, the civil rights movement, and the Second Vatican Council (Vatican II). Debates over hybrid Catholic-secular organizational partnerships and the articulation of Catholic social values with respect to workers' rights, labor laws, and abortion have accelerated. These issues have forced significant structural changes in how hospitals are run. For example, most Catholic hospitals, like secular institutions, are no longer stand-alone facilities but parts of regional or national systems governed by boards populated by large numbers of lay experts.

Questions about the changing hospital cannot be adequately understood without addressing the impact of pluralism on the secularization of social problems in twentieth-century America. Philip Gleason shows how U.S. Catholics' conceptions of their identity and their relationship to U.S. culture and institutions changed after World War II, when they adopted a "participationist version of pluralism" and denigrated 'separatism,' ethnic or otherwise."[3] The 1950s were a time when the lower and middle classes were secularizing as traditional ethnic enclaves were breaking up. Charles Morris asserts that people were "assimilating into a broader American culture that, if not quite areligious, was at least highly latitudinarian."[4]

A major thesis of this book is that as Catholic hospital leaders reacted to increased societal secularization over the course of the twentieth century, they extended their religious values in the areas of universal health care, abortion, and reproductive services, which led to tensions among the values of the Church, the government, and society. Not only do Catholic hospitals determine the types of services they offer based on Catholic religious beliefs, but they do this while supported with large pools of public funding—more than $45 billion in 2002, according to one study.[5] This support speaks to the private/public, religious/secular dichotomy that goes to the heart of the constitutional separation of church and state.

Currently, the Catholic Church owns or oversees the nation's largest group of not-for-profit health care sponsors, systems, and facilities and so exerts enormous influence on the shape of U.S. health care. As of 2009, the Catholic population was 67,117,016, or 22 percent of the total U.S. population, making it the largest single denomination in the nation. Catholic health care holdings are extensive. In 2009, more than 85 million people were assisted in 562 Catholic hospitals; 936,900 were aided in 1,643 specialized homes; and nearly 7 million were seen in 317 health care centers. Catholics own nearly three thousand social service centers and a thousand day-care and extended day-care centers. One person in six in the country is cared for in a Catholic hospital each year; and in certain areas, Catholic hospitals are the primary or only hospital available.[6] Catholic hospitals influence access to health care as well as the quality and types of services offered to both Catholics and secular communities, thus overlaying their values on a wide range of populations.

Anyone walking through the corridors of U.S. Catholic hospitals in the late nineteenth and early twentieth centuries could easily identify the hospitals' religious origins and operations.[7] Nuns in starched black-and-white habits scurried about attending to their patients and nursing duties; religious icons and paintings were present throughout the building; prayer chapels were prominently placed and identified for the benefit of all who were seeking solace or supplication; colorful patterns danced as sunlight poured through stained-glassed windows. Everything about the design and ambiance of the hospital reflected that it was much more than a medical facility; it was also a sacred place. Over the last three quarters of the twentieth century, however, the identities of Catholic hospitals went through a gradual but steady metamorphosis, not only in their appearance and ambiance, but also in their organization, management, and operations. It was a profound process of change and transformation, analogous to the crisp black and white colors of nuns' habits blending slowly into shades of gray.

In the twentieth century, Catholic hospitals attempted to fulfill religious missions to care for the sick within a commodified health delivery system. The present arrangement of U.S. hospitals includes a variety of alliances, joint ventures, networks, and other partnerships that have joined together to pool resources. This came about as a result of several circumstances in specific historical periods, an evolution Stephen M. Shortell traces. The 1920s to the

1960s witnessed several key events—the growth of third-party insurance in the 1930s; the Hospital Survey and Construction Act (Hill-Burton) in the 1940s, which led to a huge expansion in the number of hospitals; the move of hospitals from inner cities to prosperous, primarily white suburbs in the 1950s; social movements such as civil rights in the 1960s that increased care to minority groups; and Medicare and Medicaid, which expanded coverage for the elderly and poor. From the 1960s to the 1980s, investor-owned hospitals entered the hospital marketplace, when guaranteed reimbursement of costs from third-party insurers, including the government, was at its peak. From the mid 1970s through the 1980s, not-for-profit hospital systems grew, partly to counter the increasing power of investor-owned hospitals and the need to contain costs.[8] After government regulation increased in the 1980s, mergers and other forms of partnerships continued into the 1990s. Catholic hospitals negotiated these successive challenges, some as progressive, well-managed institutions, others struggling to balance their mission and business plans.

Amid external changes affecting Catholic hospitals was a change internal to U.S. Catholicism: a decline in the number of sisters and brothers in the last half of the twentieth century, the result of a drop in the number entering religious life and a huge exodus of women and men leaving their congregations after Vatican II in the 1960s. The fewer numbers entering were due to a decrease in the Catholic fertility rate, a decline in the number of Catholic schools where nuns mentored and recruited young girls, parents who were less inclined to promote the religious life when they had fewer daughters, and more ministerial Church positions open to laywomen. Some religious women left their orders because they found the life oppressing; others discovered they were not called to the religious life; and still others realized they could be ministers as laywomen rather than as religious.[9] The *Official Catholic Directory* reported 168,527 sisters and 10,473 brothers in 1960. In 1990 the number of sisters had dropped to 103,269, while brothers had decreased to 6,743.[10] In 2009, only 60,000 sisters and 4,900 brothers were in congregations. In 1980, half of Catholic hospitals' CEOs were sisters; by the 1990s the figure was 15 percent.[11] Complicating the picture was that after the 1960s, sisters and brothers began moving out of direct nursing service roles into areas such as pastoral care. At Providence Hospital in Seattle in 1960, seventeen Sisters of Providence were in residence and twenty-one were nursing students. By the end of the 1980s only six Sisters of Providence and six from other congregations worked at the hospital. Most were in pastoral care; none were nurses.[12] Consequently, sisters had less opportunity to transmit their values to people in need. At the same time, the proliferation of specialties in hospitals required more hospital personnel beyond the number that religious vocations could provide. Even had the number of vocations remained steady, the sisters and brothers would have been in the minority.[13]

Modernization, corporatization, and the disappearance of the religious communities who ran these institutions represent major changes in service organization and delivery. To understand the complexities involved, it is important to see hospitals in a market context. In January 1998, for example, the *Wall Street Journal* referred to the Daughters of Charity as "the Daughters of Currency," since their national health care system had a $2 billion investment fund and $6 billion in annual revenues. Wall Street investors were impressed.[14] Yet consolidations of secular not-for-profit and for-profit hospitals have increasingly challenged the Catholic Church's substantial presence.

As the twentieth century drew to a close, all hospitals had to balance their responsibilities to the public with their economic and political self-interests. Influenced by the pluralistic market that characterized the U.S. health care system of the twentieth century, Catholic hospitals chose to market their health care as a service. To maintain a competitive edge, they became more bureaucratized and their administrative personnel more professionalized. By the end of the century, to separate themselves from for-profit hospitals, Catholic hospital leaders were redefining their missions and recreating an ethos of religious service as they tried to recapture the public trust.[15] These were legitimate expressions of compassion and charity for the sick and uninsured. For the sisters and brothers, in particular, it was a social justice issue.

Secularization

Over the twentieth century, Catholic hospitals became more like their secular counterparts. The rise of third-party payers such as Blue Cross in the 1930s necessitated more sophisticated accounting systems. Medical advances, particularly after World War II, upped hospitals' chances to cure patients, and institutions expanded their services to accommodate the resulting increase in demand. Nuns first hired lay nurses in the early twentieth century, and the Alexian Brothers accepted laymen into their school of nursing beginning in 1939; this trend toward lay help increased after World War II.[16] Government aid expanded with the passage of the Hill-Burton Act in 1946 and Medicare and Medicaid in 1965. As the number of sisters and brothers working in hospitals decreased, lay hospital administrators were appointed, and simultaneously, charitable care ceased to be "free."[17]

Another secularizing influence came in the 1980s with the government's greater involvement in health care regulation. To cut costs, hospitals across the country reduced admissions and lengths of stay. As hospitals adopted ever more competitive business strategies, distinctions between profit and not-for-profit ownership blurred and management strategies adapted accordingly.[18] The changing health care scene affected Catholic hospitals' working environments; some personnel chose to unionize. In the process, the hospitals' public identities as institutions built on religious movements and values dimmed.

Secularization theory posits that societal advances that accompanied modernity weakened the influence of religion on Western society, a notion that has led many scholars to underestimate or disregard religion as a significant player in the twentieth century.[19] Yet James Morone asserts that religion has continued to influence the U.S. sociopolitical scene, and other critics of secularization theory note little decline in religiosity at the individual level and a push by many religions to reclaim authority in the public arena.[20] Karel Dobbelaere complicates the notion further, arguing that in the past, religious organizations could impose "the religious tradition" authoritatively, but that with increasing secularization, "it now has to be *marketed*."[21] While the Church's opposition to marketing ideas dates to the late nineteenth century, as industrial capitalism took hold, during the later twentieth century Catholic institutions tried to justify marketing on theological grounds.[22] As the focus of the debate over health care shifted, hospitals—including Catholic hospitals—became marketplace forces.[23]

The story of the transformation of Catholic hospitals sheds light not only on the broader history of U.S. hospitals but also on developments in women's reproductive health care in the United States. After abortion became legal, Catholic sisters, administrators, bishops, physicians, the laity, and policy makers interacted in an atmosphere of tension and uneasy negotiation. In the late nineteenth and early twentieth centuries, Paul Starr argues, in the hospital marketplace, ethnicity and religion, not technology, divided Catholic from lay hospitals.[24] In the later twentieth century, however, Catholic hospitals did not offer abortion and reproductive technologies, a choice that shaped the way women's health care services were provided. Reasserting their authority through the U.S. Conference of Catholic Bishops, bishops developed stricter regulations concerning partnerships of Catholic hospitals with lay hospitals that performed abortions, sterilizations, and in-vitro fertilizations, and they actively lobbied Congress against government funding for elective abortions. Because Catholic hospitals in some regions monopolized the health care delivery system, Catholic teachings could affect women's access to these services.

The Second Vatican Council

Early in the twentieth century, Catholic sisters who served as hospital owners and administrators wielded significantly greater power and authority than did most U.S. women. They were not only the administrators but also the supervisors, nurses, pharmacists, and trustees of their hospitals (see figure 1). Unlike bishops and priests, they were not part of the Church's hierarchical structure but were responsible instead to the leadership of their congregation, or order, and to its constitutions;[25] still, they remained part of a traditional and male-dominated Church.[26] After 1918, all sisters worked under restrictions codified in a Code of Canon Law that limited their interactions with the outside world. They had to report their compliance to authorities in Rome every five years and, through the 1950s, had rigid restrictions on their access to media, public meetings, and family members. Furthermore, Church edicts dating from the sixteenth century gave bishops the right to sanction enterprises in their dioceses. How sisters dealt with these sometimes conflicting authorities offers a classic example of the workings of women religious under ecclesiastical control.[27]

A renewal process, begun in the 1950s with the Sister Formation Conference that focused on the need for additional education, or formation, for congregations' specific works, had sisters by the 1960s reevaluating their dependent status.[28] They began to develop themselves spiritually and professionally. The major superiors had met in regional conferences in 1954 to organize more effective means of educating novices, culminating in 1956 with the Conference of Major Superiors of Women, an organization that brought about dramatic changes in sisters' status within the Catholic Church and U.S. society. The Conference of Major Superiors of Men was established the same year. All these groups empowered individual sisters and brothers and prepared them for their professional roles. By 1966, 65 percent of the nation's 175,000 sisters had college degrees.[29] In 1971, the Conference of Major Superiors of Women changed its name to the Leadership Conference of Women Religious, a signal of the changing understanding of women's roles in the Church. The sisters and brothers who participated in these conferences were unique in their preparation, and the progressive reforms they pushed caused some painful self-examination in their religious communities and dismay on the part of some lay Catholics.[30]

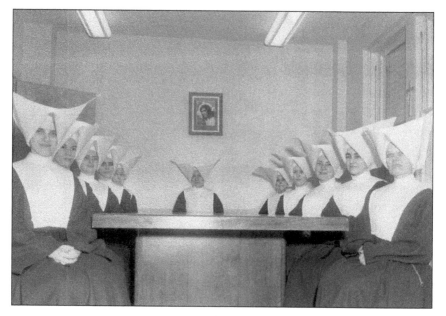

Figure 1 Seton Daughters of Charity in boardroom, Austin, Texas, ca. mid-1950s. These sisters comprised the Board of Trustees.

Courtesy Seton Family of Hospitals, Archives Division, Austin, Texas.

One of the most important events in recent world history, the Second Vatican Council, Vatican II, met from 1962 to 1965. Its significance, as well as its influence on health care and policy, are as yet poorly understood by U.S. historians. Vatican II changed how Catholic religious orders viewed their vocations and the Church itself and produced a paradigmatic shift for Catholic hospitals: leadership roles in Catholic institutions were opened to the laity.

Aggiornamento, or change and adaptation to meet the needs of the times, was one of the key terms used during the Council. The Council document most often linked with *aggiornamento* is *Gaudium et Spes* (Joy and Hope), or the Pastoral Constitution on the Church in the Modern World, which declared that all people, including laymen and women, have distinctive missions in the Church rather than being mere "helpers of the hierarchy."[31] As John McGreevy argues, the Second Council's emphasis on human dignity and justice, as opposed to charity, prompted a worldwide reassessment of Catholic social policy that led institutional Catholicism to become an international defender of human rights. Social justice efforts on the part of religious orders, such as going out into the world to care for the poor and dispossessed, received greater emphasis.[32] Religious congregations held meetings to redefine their governance and ministry and renewed their commitment to the poor and oppressed.

As one sister stated: "Vatican II took us out of the ghettos and into ecology, feminism and justice in the world. . . . The Vatican still has a difficult time accepting that."[33] As a result of Vatican II, individual nuns could confer with their congregation's administrators about where they would work rather than simply accept appointments, a change that continued to cause some tensions within congregations. Some sisters stated that when they entered an order, they committed themselves to their congregation's work, regardless of where they were sent. Others now opted for areas of service of their own choosing. As the recorder noted at a 1971 meeting of the Sisters of Saint Joseph of Rochester: "The old-time 'slot-filling' assignment still seem[ed] to be a concept in the minds of some Sisters in spite of the opportunities given year after year for the individual to make recommendations concerning her personal assignment."[34] These changes were factors in a congregation's ability to continue to staff hospitals, for as congregations reevaluated Church, educational, and health care institutions, some relinquished their hospitals altogether to focus on social justice issues in other ways.[35]

With the election of Pope John Paul II in 1978, however, the tendency toward uniformity and control by the Vatican made a comeback, replacing the more collegial model that had developed after Vatican II. This trend coincided with a conservative religious movement across the United States. The U.S. Catholic Church reasserted male supremacy, again denounced abortion and artificial birth control, and criticized priests and sisters who held public office.[36] Coupled with sisters' decreasing numbers, this led to a decline in their influence in the overall hospital market. However, in some parts of the country individual sisters maintained power over their institutions, while in others they lost control over hospital operations but gained influence as members of boards of directors and officers in the Catholic Health Association.

Catholic Religious Congregations and Hospitals

Catholic religious congregations' hospitals reflect the changes in the U.S. health care setting over the twentieth century. Voluntary hospitals such as Catholic institutions began as private, not-for-profit facilities that relied on patient fees and donations for support. These institutions developed with distinct identities according to place, ethnicity, economics, race, education, and unionization. The Sisters of Charity began staffing an infirmary at the University of Maryland in 1823; thereafter, many different religious congregations opened hospitals during epidemics and war, in cities and frontier outposts, and in railroad and mining camps. Madame Emile Tavernier Gamelin, SP, established the Sisters of Providence in Montreal, Quebec, Canada, in 1843 in response to a cholera epidemic.[37] In 1856, Mother Joseph Pariseau, SP, and four other Sisters of Providence arrived in Vancouver, Washington Territory, and eventually established many hospitals in the Northwest. Unlike U.S. congregations in the late nineteenth century that were receiving hundreds of Irish women or daughters of Irish immigrants, the Sisters of Providence attracted few Irish and maintained their French-Canadian identity well into the 1930s, as Sioban Nelson recounts, writing their chronicles in French through that period. Nurtured by the Montreal motherhouse, they continued to receive women recruits from Quebec until 1944.[38]

Ten years after the Sisters of Providence arrived in Vancouver, in 1866 Brother Bonaventure Thelan, CFA, established a hospital in Chicago, confirming a long tradition of caring for the poor and destitute among the Alexian Brothers. The brothers began as a group of nonliterate men who organized in Germany and the Low Countries in the early fourteenth century to bury the dead during the height of the catastrophic Black Death, or bubonic plague. By the seventeenth century, they were tending to a variety of social outsiders, such as criminals and the mentally ill. In the nineteenth century the Alexian Brothers adopted the same tradition women's religious nursing orders had, establishing hospitals and providing nursing care in many countries.[39]

While many religious orders of men nursed in the medieval period, in the seventeenth-century Saint Vincent de Paul made religious women more prevalent in nursing when he and Saint Louise de Marillac established the Daughters of Charity in France in 1633.[40] Unlike the cloistered women's communities that participated primarily in contemplative prayer, the Daughters cared for the sick by living among people whom society had abandoned. Nearly two centuries later, in 1809, the American Elizabeth Ann Seton founded the Sisters of Charity of Saint Joseph in Emmitsburg, Maryland. In 1850, the Emmitsburg community united with the international Daughters of Charity based in Paris, becoming the first U.S. community of the Daughters of Charity of Saint Vincent de Paul.[41] The Daughters shared the belief of many bishops that Catholic hospitals were the most effective tools of evangelization in areas where the Church was not well known; between 1892 and 1909, they opened hospitals in Texas and other areas in the South.

Many of the U.S. Daughters of Charity had Irish backgrounds, as did the congregation founded by Catherine McAuley in Dublin, in 1831, the Sisters of Mercy, who arrived in the United States in 1843 with a long history of visiting the sick poor in their homes in Ireland. The Irish sisters began by caring for people stricken with typhus and cholera; then, under the direction of Mother Frances Warde, in 1847 they established the first hospital in Pittsburgh. A year earlier, with Mother Frances Warde's guidance, five Irish sisters, including Agatha O'Brien as superior, had traveled from Pittsburgh to Chicago, where in 1851 they took over the city's makeshift hospital; this became Mercy Hospital, the first chartered hospital in Chicago.[42]

Catholic Hospitals and General Hospital History

Sisters and brothers reframed themselves in the last half of the twentieth century as they used their hospital ministry as an avenue for social justice. In the process, they carved out social and political territory through negotiations with medical and nursing personnel, secular organizations, policy strategists, unions, the federal government, and the public. They faced changing beliefs about traditional provision of charity to the deserving poor versus the rights of all for health care. Vast biomedical changes were occurring along with national economic upheaval, a world war followed by the cold war, the civil rights movement, and the role of very large private and public actors in the hospital marketplace.

U.S. hospitals grew from 4,359 in 1909 to 6,852 in 1928, an increase of 57 percent. By the late 1920s, changes in medical technology included x-rays, laboratories, and aseptic surgery. In the decade after 1928, hospitals steadily declined in number, and occupancy rates decreased during the early years of the Great Depression.[43] The situation improved in the late 1930s, as private hospital insurance plans such as Blue Cross became more popular and accounted for a greater percentage of hospital financing; the American Hospital Association (AHA) began approving Blue Cross plans in 1937. Health insurance remedied much of the financial risk hospitals took, and they profited from the start. After 1938, not only did the number of both government and nongovernment hospitals increase, but also they expanded their facilities. By 1941, the number of beds had risen more than 300 percent since 1909, mainly in voluntary and government hospitals. Proprietary, or for-profit, hospitals accounted for only 4 percent of the total. The number of hospital beds in the 1940s continued to outstrip population growth.[44]

A surge of demand for hospitals occurred after World War II as advances in science and technology offered improved prospects of care. Government aid became increasingly important, with huge amounts of money going to hospital enterprises in the form of Hill-Burton grants. At the 1946 Catholic Hospital Association (CHA) convention, association president Rev. Alphonse Schwitalla told the 3,500 delegates, mostly nuns who were superintendents or supervisors of Catholic hospitals, of the expansion plans of 552 Catholic hospitals, including $8,880,000 to be spent by hospitals in the Far West.[45]

Voluntary-hospital insurance plans expanded rapidly, from 9 percent of the population in 1940 to 71.4 percent in 1965.[46] The 685 U.S. Catholic hospitals in 1945 had a bed capacity of 87,171; by 1960, 800 Catholic hospitals had 136,689 beds.[47] Between 1960 and 1970, the number of patients treated annually in Catholic hospitals nearly doubled. By 2000, however, reflecting the era of hospital mergers, Catholic hospitals decreased in number while patient admissions continued to grow (see table 1.1).

After Medicare and Medicaid passed in 1965, hospitals' increased incomes enabled them, once again, to expand; indeed, the more expenditures hospitals incurred, the more reimbursement they received from the government. Medicare and Medicaid, as Rosemary Stevens asserts, "fed the market enthusiasm of the 1970s. It was now permissible (indeed admirable) for voluntary hospitals to post a surplus, indicating effective management." The AHA relabeled voluntary institutions "not for profit" rather than "nonprofit," and proprietary hospitals "for profit" or "investor owned."[48]

Table 1.1   **Growth of Catholic Hospitals and Schools of Nursing, 1945–2000**

Year	Hospitals	Bed capacity	Patients treated annually	Schools of nursing	Nursing students
1945	685	87,171	3,290,821	n.a.	n.a.
1950	739	96,349	4,567,934	367	30,211
1960	808	136,689	12,819,798	347	34,395
1970	764	155,235	21,015,589	260	23,875
1980	633	166,998	34,252,953	121	19,423
1990	641	n.a.	43,407,335	n.a.	n.a.
2000	593	n.a.	77,006,804	n.a.	n.a.

Source: *Official Catholic Directory* (New York: P. J. Kenedy and Sons).

Nursing Education

In the mid-twentieth century, nursing education began to move from three-year hospital-based diploma programs to four-year baccalaureate schools in U.S. colleges and universities, and Catholic schools followed this path (see table 1.1). University degree programs gained popularity in the 1930s and 1940s, and for the first time, despite many years of experience in teaching and nursing, sisters and brothers felt they were inferior professionally to college-educated nurses. Most of the young sisters and brothers in the 1930s, 1940s, and 1950s were assigned to their congregation's hospitals before completing their diplomas in nursing. Yet some of the Sisters of Mercy in Chicago and the Sisters of Providence in Seattle were able to take university courses in the 1930s and 1940s.[49] The Sister Formation Conference in the 1950s benefited sisters and brothers in nursing as well as those in education. Not without struggle, many were able to finish their nursing degrees before starting full-time employment.[50] After the Sister Formation program, for example, Sister Karin Dufault, SP, of the Sisters of Providence, graduated from Seattle University with a bachelor of science in nursing, later completed her master's and doctorate in nursing with a specialty in oncology and the elderly, and eventually chaired the CHA board of trustees.[51]

As with their other ministries, Catholic religious communities opened and closed schools of nursing in response to changing trends and circumstances. All the hospitals in this study established schools of nursing and eventually relocated from hospital-owned programs to private and public baccalaureate schools. The Alexian Brothers Hospital School of Nursing for men incorporated in 1898. While many of the lay nursing staff were obtaining advanced degrees in the 1950s, the Alexian Brothers were not allowed to do so until the late 1950s and early 1960s. The last class graduated in 1969 after baccalaureate programs became available in Chicago.[52] In Seattle, Providence Hospital School of Nursing opened in 1907; the entire nursing collegiate program was transferred to Seattle College (a Jesuit institution) in 1941, with clinical experiences offered at Providence Hospital.[53] The Daughters of Charity established Seton Hospital's School of Nursing in Austin in 1902. By 1965 they had nearly three hundred hospital affiliations across the country. That year, after a downward trend in the number of diploma programs and a shift toward associate and baccalaureate schools, the Daughters began closing their diploma schools; the exceptions were six programs that lasted into the 1980s and 1990s. Seton's program eventually affiliated with the University of Texas baccalaureate program.[54]

In 1889 in Chicago, the Sisters of Mercy began Mercy Training School for Nurses as a three-year diploma program, the first Catholic nursing school in Illinois and the order's first in the country. In 1905, the sisters affiliated the School of Nursing with Northwestern University. Mercy leaders were well aware of the Goldmark Report of 1923 that had criticized the typical training school and encouraged collegiate programs of nursing education. Both Catholic and non-Catholic schools were slow to follow the report's recommendations, and not until 1935 did Mercy Hospital Training School affiliate with the sisters' own Saint Francis Xavier College for Women, where women could obtain a bachelor of science degree in nursing. Students who opted for the three-year diploma program received a graduate nurse certificate. By 1938, most students were entering the degree program. During the Great Depression, however, the sisters felt they needed students from the diploma school to help staff the hospital, and they retained that program until 1959 (see figure 2).[55]

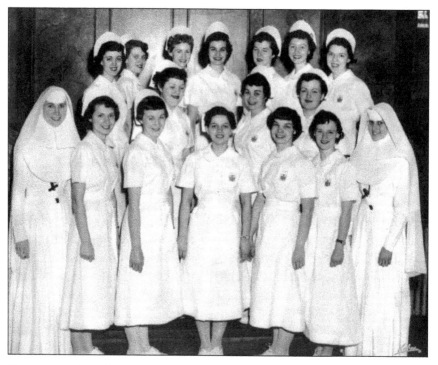

Figure 2   Class of 1956, Mercy School of Nursing, Saint Xavier College, Chicago, Illinois.

Courtesy Mercy Hospital and Medical Center Archives, Chicago, Illinois.

Mercy Hospital School of Nursing in Pittsburgh is one of the few nursing diploma programs still in existence. The Sisters of Mercy established it in 1893, and from 1899 to 1934, they also supported a school for men to meet increased industrial demands for care of injured male employees. In 1926, Mercy School of Nursing began offering an affiliation with Duquesne University to obtain a bachelor of science degree in nursing. Students received a diploma after completing three years of nursing courses at Mercy, then went on to two additional years at Duquesne for their bachelor's. Mercy's school affiliated with the sisters' own Mount Mercy College (now Carlow) for a bachelor of science in nursing in 1948, but the hospital still supports its diploma program.[56]

As insurance companies gained influence during the 1950s, they also helped dismantle diploma nursing programs by refusing to allow hospitals to include school costs as patient expenses. By the 1960s diploma programs were becoming financial burdens to hospitals. In addition, after 1965, federal dollars were available for nursing education, which supported its expansion into higher education. The number of Catholic schools by 1980 was one-third that in 1950. Furthermore, as hospital diploma programs closed and nursing students no longer provided the institutions with cheap labor, hospitals hired graduate nurses, whose salaries significantly increased costs.[57]

Growth of Health Care Systems

In 1970, the American Hospital Association listed 7,123 hospitals in the United States, up 247 from 1960. A major shift had occurred in hospital clientele during this decade: the number of beds in federal, psychiatric, tuberculosis, and other long-term care facilities had declined, while, aided by government funding, beds in community hospitals increased by 32.7 percent. Controlled by community leaders, these nonfederal, short-term general hospitals were linked to local physicians to meet community needs. They represented 82.3 percent of all hospitals, contained more than half of all hospital beds, and had 92.1 percent of all admissions.[58]

For all the government support from Medicare and Medicaid, the cost of hospital care grew even faster. By the 1970s, Catholic hospitals, like others, offered more comprehensive and complex services, such as open-heart surgery, dialysis, radioisotope procedures, social work services, and in-house psychiatric facilities. Intensive care units increased and machines became ever more prevalent.[59] Demand for capital increased as more money was needed to start new projects and replace deteriorating buildings and equipment. "This was not merely a matter of institutional self-interest," Stevens points out. "Hospitals had a public mandate—even a social duty—to expand, rebuild, and re-equip."[60] But these changes, along with new treatments and technologies, contributed to escalating in-patient hospital costs that led to federal wage and price controls in 1971. In 1975, at Mercy Hospital in Chicago, the Business Office worked with patients who did not have health insurance coverage to ensure their bills were paid, helping them secure a bank loan, apply for public aid assistance, or sign a promissory note. "We do not serve in order to collect money," stated the director of admissions, "but we must collect money in order to serve."[61]

In the 1980s the balance of power in health care institutions shifted from producers to organized purchasers of care. Indeed, the years after 1965 and the passage of Medicare and Medicaid were pivotal for everyone in health care, not only because of increased government regulation but also because of lucrative profits. In response, Medicare incorporated a prospective payment system in 1983 that radically changed its reimbursements. Federal programs went from paying all costs, to paying what costs should be, to paying a preset fee for a specific illness in the form of Diagnostic Related Groups, or DRGs. The AHA and the CHA requested a delay in implementing the national rates because the financial impact would be so severe on their member hospitals, submitting a proposal of their own that the Health Care Financing Administration did not think gave hospitals enough incentive to change their behavior.[62] Meanwhile, a growing segment of the U.S. population was either unemployed or working in low-paying jobs, could not afford hospital care, and did not qualify for federal assistance.[63]

For-profit hospital networks, increasing since the early 1970s, became much more central in the 1980s, representing competition that made smaller not-for-profit institutions more vulnerable. More than six hundred community hospitals closed, including some Catholic ones.[64] In response, surviving Catholic hospitals and other not-for-profit institutions began forming larger hospital systems, marking a significant change in the voluntary hospital arena. The resulting multihospital systems were corporate entities that owned or operated more than one hospital. Catholic religious congregations that historically had been autonomous and separately incorporated became major actors in the multihospital system movement.[65]

In fact, Catholic health care congregations possessed characteristics that lent themselves to success in forming systems, as Sister Mary Maurita Sengelaub, RSM, former executive director of the CHA, pointed out. The vast majority were owned by Catholic religious congregations, the remainder by a diocese. Each group was accustomed to operating more than one hospital or health care institution at a time. For example, in 1978, forty-five of approximately two hundred religious congregations operated 75 percent of Catholic acute care hospitals, and each sponsored four or more hospitals. The remaining congregations sponsored from one to four hospitals each. This background increased Catholic congregations' potential for success as they developed their own systems and proved a major strength for them in the expanding hospital marketplace.[66]

A systems approach created unique opportunities for sisters and brothers. They could be trustees at the system's corporate and local boards, and they could serve as consultants, monitoring patient services, exercising stewardship, and guiding hospital philosophy, mission, and values.[67] As members of local boards, they could still participate in hospital decisions, which rested with local boards of directors accountable to the health system office. In large medical centers, a system representative served on the local board, and the system would be involved on any major strategic initiative, but the local board made the decision. Sponsoring organizations were the religious congregations themselves, which reserved powers spelled out in the bylaws of each institution. The congregation's leaders exercised their reserved powers when approving the mission, selling hospitals, and purchasing a certain amount of goods or property. Sisters and brothers who served on boards of directors were members of the sponsoring congregation but had no more authority than any other board member.[68]

Religious congregations collaborated in various ways. The Sisters of Mercy, for example, had hospitals that were independent of each other in numerous regions, or provinces. Between 1965 and 1975, however, the Detroit Province established five multiunit corporations in Michigan, Indiana, and Iowa. Similarly, in 1986 the Daughters of Charity of Saint Vincent de Paul joined their five geographic areas and two regional systems to become the country's largest not-for-profit health care system. To maintain a Catholic health care presence in a community, some Catholic hospitals participated in mergers or acquisitions even when market forces were unfavorable. Other mergers occurred between Catholic and non-Catholic not-for-profit and even for-profit systems. By 1985 there were 91 Catholic health care systems out of a total of 268. As large-scale corporate enterprises grew, 553 Catholic hospitals belonged to a multihospital system.[69] But questions remained about how to deal with the image of Catholic health care as big business. And was it a desirable development?

In 1984, the president of the American Hospital Association asserted that not-for-profit and government hospitals looked more and more like "their for-profit counterparts, because they basically are being financed from the capital expenditure side by invested money and by borrowed money, and both sources expect a return on the money."[70] Many religious congregations questioned the morality of the trend toward corporate models that emphasized secular values, given their history of care for the poor as their institutions' founding principle. In the 1980s, concern increased that priorities were not the health and medical needs of the poor. In 1982, bishops questioned the very existence of Catholic hospitals if they could not extend service to the poor and elderly. Hospital chief executives concurred. All agreed that commitment to the poor was the key to Catholic identity.[71]

Yet religious congregations had to weigh the cost of rigidly adhering to mission principles against compromising these principles to stay in business so they could serve people in need. In some circles, this compromise was unacceptable, but Catholic congregations lived in a secular world, serving people of all faiths and of none at all. While they made no compromises with their personal Catholic faith, religious congregations that stayed in the hospital business operated in the gray area of reconciliation between rigid adherence to Catholic ideals and a strictly business approach. At the same time, these businesswomen and businessmen maintained a strong sense of mission.

The struggle to find the proper balance between market and mission was evident in 1987 at the CHA annual meeting. Delegates called for a "rededication" to the health care ministry, described as "the business of being holy, the business of being a community, and the business of caring for people."[72] In addition to the auspicious use of the term "rededication," notably missing was a commitment to pursue business principles that fostered success and growth in the competitive hospital marketplace. From that significant omission, one can conclude that Catholic health care leaders felt the balance between market and mission had drifted too close to the business spectrum and too far from the original mission of serving all in need, regardless of financial circumstances.

Yet adhering to the mission of serving the poor while balancing economic needs became an even greater challenge as total national spending on health care continued to rise, despite government and private initiatives to decrease costs. In 1988, for example, health spending increased 10.4 percent over 1987 and accounted for 11.1 percent of the gross national product. As a result, cost containment became a major issue in the 1990s.[73]

Hospital administrators across the country responded by streamlining their operations and restructuring through mergers—190 between 1990 and 1996.[74] Consolidation of religious hospitals increased; in some areas, Catholic health care systems became the largest employers. For example, the St. Louis–based Daughters of Charity in the early 1990s employed seventy-one thousand workers and had approximately $4 billion in assets. These employment and financial data reveal how important Catholic health care systems had become to the trillion-dollar national health care industry. Catholic health care had, indeed, become a competitive industry. As Arthur Jones argues, while individual hospitals maintained charitable care and community involvement as part of their mission, they were as "cost conscious and dollar-driven as their secular counterparts."[75] The push for profits led to replacing some skilled nursing staff with aides, shorter hospital stays, and more care provided outside hospitals. In the private sector, third-party payers continued to take an active role in managing hospital costs. Health maintenance organizations that contracted with a network of providers for discounted prices increased in importance.

Uncompensated Care

For both Catholic and non-Catholic hospitals, changes in the health care system raised concerns about care for the uninsured. Resources for care to the medically indigent are typically measured by uncompensated care costs, that is, the combined cost of charity care and bad debt, which for private hospitals rose during the 1980s but remained stable in the 1990s.[76] To maintain their missions, including funding for uncompensated care, all hospitals historically have either engaged in cost shifting (offsetting the cost of unpaid care for one group by charging more to another) or accepted lower profit margins. They have also drawn on private philanthropy and public sources such as tax revenues, uncompensated care pools, or disproportionate-share adjustments in Medicare and Medicaid.[77] From the late 1980s into the early 1990s, hospital budget balancing focused on cost shifting. For those with private insurance, the result was higher premiums. Below-cost public payers such as Medicare and Medicaid paid less for services, and they and the uninsured benefited at private payers' expense. This system ensured coverage for uncompensated care and allowed hospitals to carry out their missions of teaching, research, or, in the case of Catholic hospitals, charity care.

With the growth of managed care in the mid 1990s, however, as market power shifted away from hospitals toward managed care companies, hospitals were less able to use this cost-shifting strategy. They now had to negotiate prices with private insurance companies, which were no longer willing to pay higher hospital prices. Some states in these years developed alternative mechanisms to help fund hospitals that provided high levels of uncompensated care.[78]

Hospital Trends, 1995

In 1995, the hospitals in the four cities highlighted in this book—Austin, Chicago, Pittsburgh, and Seattle—reflected the nationwide decline in admissions, daily census, and occupancy rates, as well as an increase in outpatient visits from previous years (see table 1.2).[79] Lengths of stay also declined all over the country to an average of 6.5 days. Seattle hospitals, where managed care had penetrated, were experiencing shorter lengths of stay, as were those in Austin. Pittsburgh and Chicago hospitals reported longer stays for varied reasons, which might include case mix and medical practice styles. They also were located in large urban areas, and both had long-standing outpatient clinics that employed large numbers of medical residents and interns.

The average daily census and occupancy rates in the cities' hospitals ranged from 65 to 73 percent, indicating large numbers of empty beds in all four areas. Hospital costs were highest in Seattle, likely because of unionization and a higher cost of living. For-profit hospitals had penetrated heavily into Austin, and fierce competition along with lower labor costs could account for the lower expenses there. The presence in Austin of the Columbia/Hospital Corporation of America chain, the largest for-profit hospital group in the country, significantly affected the Daughters of Charity's competitive strategies.

At the same time, the midnineties, 40.3 million people in the United States were uninsured. Regional variations were apparent; for example, 27 percent of the Texas population was uninsured. The continuing rise in the uninsured affected community hospitals, which saw an increase in emergency room visits. While cities such as Chicago benefited from state supplements to hospitals to offset uncompensated care costs, greater emergency room use could still be costly.[80] The Balanced Budget Act of 1997 decreased Medicare payments to hospitals by $115 billion over five years, and when Medicare did not cover hospital costs, the number of in-patient admissions plunged. While some hospitals admitted fewer patients, others did not necessarily decrease the number of Medicare admissions but rather cut costs by discharging people sooner.[81]

Table 1.2 **Hospital Characteristics in Selected Cities, 1995**

	Chicago	Austin	Seattle	Pittsburgh
Utilization				
Hospitals	43	8	9	21
Beds	12,559	1,540	2,648	7,794
Admissions	442,077	72,853	119,049	276,575
Inpatient days	2,992,211	363,146	638,766	2,080,699
Average daily census (occupancy rate)	8,219 (65%)	1,024 (67%)	1,751 (66%)	5,700 (73%)
Average stay (days)	6.8	5.0	5.4	7.5
Outpatients				
ER	1,145,419	213,505	350,256	588,083
Total	5,634,795	596,581	2,367,237	3,294,748
Expenses				
Adjusted cost per admission	$8,389.90	$5,518.66	$9,466.32	$9,122.53
Adjusted cost per inpatient day	$1,242.43	$1,108.25	$1,768.84	$1,230.49
Payroll (in thousands)	$2,354,991	$212,574	$734,427	$1,357,423
Employee benefits (in thousands)	$460,223	$38,527	$169,512	$305,157

Source: *1995 Annual Survey of Hospitals* (Chicago: American Hospital Association, 1996).

By the end of the 1990s, most Catholic hospitals, like their secular counterparts, were part of large regional or multistate systems.[82] While increased competition had pressured many hospitals to reduce their operating costs, empirical evidence was showing that hospital mergers, ostensibly undertaken to reduce competition, were leading to price increases at all the merging institutions, profit and not-for-profit.[83] As hospitals became more willing to raise prices to exploit market power, antitrust regulators entered the picture to approve the mergers. All hospitals were increasingly vulnerable to federal regulation, and Catholic hospitals, like others, had to submit plans for future consolidation for approval.[84]

In summary, in the last half of the twentieth century, Catholic hospitals had to find new ways to operate in a changed, secularized society. Their power structures shifted, and their employees and local communities perceived them in new ways. As religious congregations dealt with these changes, they faced more questions. Would the current trend in larger systems lead to a Catholic health care ministry that was too large and too corporate? Would systems stray too far from the congregation's special ministry to the poor? What were the roles of sisters and brothers in health care and in the ongoing Catholic identity of their hospitals?

Chapter 2

A Precarious Economic Scene

The "economic scene was precarious," the political scene "hyperactive," and "the religious scene fraught with confusion and anxiety," wrote the Providence Hospital chronicler in Seattle, Washington, on June 30, 1970, regarding the many changes that had stirred unrest among the sisters as hospital leaders.[1] Of course, this was the seventies, a decade that saw those very social conditions in the United States. But for Catholics in particular, the ecclesiastical edicts of Vatican II had brought about significant and often disruptive cultural changes, and with the sharp dropoff in numbers of new priests, brothers, and sisters, more and more non-Catholics were handling the day-to-day operations of Catholic institutions.

While the U.S. market-oriented system seemed poorly suited to Catholic goals of health care—to provide quality care for all with compassion and respect regardless of ability to pay—many Catholic hospitals managed to survive.[2] Among them, Providence Hospital, the Sisters of Providence institution in Seattle; the Alexian Brothers Hospital in Chicago; the Daughters of Charity's Seton Hospital in Austin; and the Sisters of Mercy's hospitals in Pittsburgh and Chicago by 2000 had each created a new identity based on commitment to promoting and defending human dignity, with special attention to the poor and underserved.

Keeping Some Facilities, Closing Others

In the early 1990s, many states began experiments in managed care and became more open to calls for universal health care coverage. In Washington,

Catholic institutions adopted strategies that involved hospital-to-hospital and hospital-to-physician collaborations. They formed networks with physicians, insurers, and other community agencies; offered ambulatory care centers for acute care services; established hospice, home health, and psychiatric services, and rehabilitation for the chronically ill; and contracted with managed care and other insurance plans.[3] As the year 1995 began, however, a new Republican majority in Congress aimed to decrease government spending and especially targeted a cut in the Medicare budget. At the state level, Republicans also gained power; they held thirty state governorships, including Washington's. That year, the Republicans in the Washington State Legislature cut back on mandates for universal coverage, significantly affecting Providence Medical Center in Seattle, founded in 1877 as Providence Hospital.

One of the Sisters of Providence's largest institutions, Providence Hospital went through the same difficulties other hospitals suffered during the Great Depression and World War II, when it experienced a steady decline of physicians and nurses, although the U.S. Cadet Nurse Corps, an organization Congress established to fill the wartime nursing shortage, eased the situation. After the war, the sisters borrowed money, obtained government funding, and used community fundraisers to expand their hospital in 1949, 1962, and 1965. After Medicare and Medicaid entered the picture, bureaucratic problems mounted, requiring personnel with greater expertise in business principles. The sisters hired Richard J. Borsini as Providence Hospital's first lay administrator in 1967.[4]

Throughout the 1960s, the hospital's occupancy rates remained high. By 1970, Medicare paid for 24 percent of total admissions, with Medicaid paying only 4 percent. Providence expanded early in the decade into the profitable area of cardiac care and also established itself as a center for hospice, honoring the sisters' continued dedication to attending to the spiritual as well as the physical needs of dying patients. Rather than adopt the in-patient cost-cutting going on in hospitals across the country, the sisters began planning for an alternative birthing facility and ambulatory surgery department to generate more revenue.

In 1974, the Health Resources and Development Act created state certificate of need laws, which Washington, along with other states, adopted, requiring hospitals to justify additions and major expenditures. Providence leaders applied to the Washington State Hospital Commission for a certificate of need for a new hospital wing and a computerized tomography scanner, a detailed and lengthy process that ended in approval and allowed them

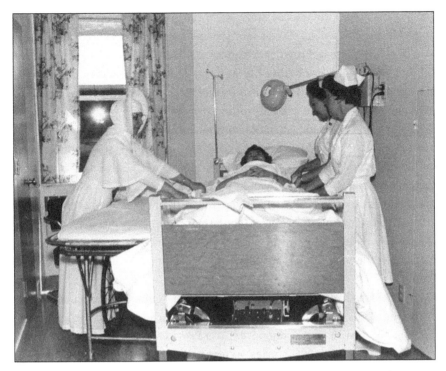

Figure 3 Sister Gilberte Parent, SP, nursing supervisor, and lay nurses with patient, Seattle, Washington, ca. 1963.

Photo # 56.C21.72, Providence Seattle Medical Center, Providence Archives, Mother Joseph Province, Seattle, Washington.

to begin the first phase of a new building project for a heart center, critical care units, and emergency and family practice departments. To take over the fund-raising, the Providence Foundation of Seattle was formed. In 1979 the hospital was renamed Providence Medical Center. A Planned Giving Committee was established in the 1980s to increase commitments through wills, bequests, trusts, and insurance gifts.[5]

The second and third building phases had to be postponed, however, in light of the economic recession of the 1980s. In Washington, a depressed timber industry raised Seattle's unemployment rate, which combined with increasing hospital costs and cuts in social service funds to produce a lower patient census than projected. By then, Providence was serving a large Medicaid population, and the government had doubled the time it took to pay hospitals for a Medicaid patient, now eighty-three days; cash-flow problems resulted. In

1983, the hospital provided $13 million in uncompensated care and was over budget due to low census, larger salaries, and increased supply costs.[6]

To counter losses, Providence contracted in 1987 to care for Pacific Medical Center's clients—including a large group of federal defense contractors—at a negotiated discount. The deal boosted admissions, and Providence readily obtained a certificate of need to restart the next phases of its construction and renovation program. At the same time, as prospective payment systems and insurance companies pressed hospitals to decrease inpatient admissions, outpatient volume at Providence increased significantly. Alternative delivery systems such as Health Maintenance Organizations (HMOs) and Preferred Provider Organizations (PPOs) had expanded their operations in the Seattle area. With increasing government regulations to cut costs, the average length of stay at Providence decreased; consequently, in 1988 the medical center lost money. On the plus side of the ledger, the Providence Foundation brought in $847,000.[7]

As debates over market ideas in health care gained prominence in the 1970s and 1980s, hospital ethics committees began addressing issues of competition and health care economics.[8] At a Providence Medical Morals Committee conference in 1986, a priest expressed his view that competition was "evil," born of the "passion for power." A sister responded that competition was a reality in health care, but that Providence could fulfill its mission without having to engage in fierce competition with other hospitals.[9] In making these statements, both speakers mistakenly assumed that other groups working in health care shared their basic ideals, but health care participants such as insurance companies, expanding for-profit hospitals, and government regulatory agencies had goals based on market perspectives. Hence the sisters could not ignore the notion of competition, since their hospitals could not survive if they did not pay attention to the market. Historically, Catholic sisters had tried to provide the best possible care, buy the best supplies, hire the best physicians, develop services that both physicians and the community wanted, and advertise their high-quality products—all tools of the market.[10] Although some Catholic leaders thought they could operate from idealism, it was not possible in the hospital market of the 1980s.

By the end of 1987, marketing had emerged as an important component of hospital planning, and one of Providence Medical Center's goals was to "increase market share in selected inpatient and outpatient services." That year the hospital chronicler admitted that competition was a reality in Seattle with its oversupply of hospitals.[11] Providers had to compete to attract doctors, businesses, and consumers. Some observers accused the sisters of being hypocritical for participating in these activities; others saw them as pragmatic as they tried to keep the hospital solvent. To keep the sisters' religious mission prominent, a new publicity campaign in the 1980s highlighted the nuns' traditional mission to provide health care to all, regardless of ability to pay. Programs focused on such topics as "Do our decisions reflect our mission?" Sisters themselves played key roles, educating employees about the basic tenets of their philosophy and mentoring future leaders. To educate the lay leadership, hospital leaders invited candidates running for various state offices to meet with the hospital's Legislative Affairs Committee to make sure they understood the nuns' mission.[12]

In 1991, the governance of the hospital corporation reorganized, separating the sisters' Provincial Council from governance of the health system: the Provincial Council was no longer the board of directors of the hospital, and the provincial superior was no longer the designated chair of the board. However, the superior and council members were corporate members who could appoint those who served on the board. Furthermore, some members of the council were still board members along with other religious and lay people, and a Sister of Providence could still be chair. In 2000, while there were only two Sisters of Providence working at the hospital, Sister Karin Dufault, SP, held the influential chair of the board of directors.[13]

As sisters' presence dwindled over the latter half of the twentieth century, other kinds of problems arose. Employees expressed concern about communication between themselves and lay administrators and managers. As a result, in 1991 lay hospital leaders began efforts to increase the visibility of the administration. At the same time, cost-saving measures and a cutback of twenty-four managerial nursing positions improved the economic status of Providence. Although at the cost of nurses, by 1992 Providence Medical Center was financially stable.[14]

Management considered the greatest challenge facing them in the 1990s to be health care reform at the state and national levels. As an example, in 1991, hospital leaders in the state, physicians, other Sisters of Providence institutions, and Providence Medical Center employees vigorously opposed Washington State's Initiative 119, which would have allowed assisted suicide. The bill did not pass.[15] More important for Providence's survival, however, was its commitment to the state's ill-fated 1993 health care reform plan that was to guarantee health coverage to all residents; a Democrat-controlled state legislature passed the Health Services Act that provided, among other benefits, a system of individual and employer mandates to create universal coverage. To put Providence in a good position to offer businesses an efficient medical care package, the hospital's leaders invested in an extensive network of primary care clinics. They also moved toward greater integration with local physicians and started a health insurance plan.[16] The hospital had a steady increase in outpatient surgery; a solid system of primary care clinics and home care and hospice services; and a new skilled nursing facility. Providence now held what hospital leaders thought would be a strong strategic position to participate in a health care delivery system based on managed care.[17]

But in 1995, a new conservative administration at the state level repealed some elements of the Health Services Act, including mandates for universal coverage. Had the mandates continued, Providence would have capitalized on the regulated managed care system for which it had prepared; instead, it lost millions of dollars.

Two years earlier, declines in admissions had combined with a decrease in in-patient lengths of stay to force Providence to lay off eighty workers, including registered nurses and twenty people in management positions, to eliminate time-and-a-half twelve-hour weekend shifts, and to hire more nursing assistants. Now the Center's health insurance plan closed, as did some of its clinics. Competition in Seattle had, indeed, been fierce. Swedish Medical Center scooped up Providence's contract with Pacific Medical Center and, with advertisements emphasizing Swedish's specialty practice, lured several heart surgeons away from Providence. Their leaving supported other specialty physicians' beliefs that Providence's commitment to primary care was at their expense. The loss of the surgeons was a major blow: 25 percent of Providence's revenue came from heart surgeries. The newly renamed Providence Seattle Medical Center now lost 20 percent of its patient volume from its most productive service.[18]

As the hospital channeled funds into primary care, its physical plant was deteriorating, and Providence Medical Group's below-budget performance in 1999 resulted in the closure of even more clinics. Low patient volumes in the hospital now necessitated layoffs of nearly four hundred full-time employees. Further complicating the picture, the University of Washington/Northwest Hospital obtained a certificate of need for open-heart surgery. Charity care continued at Providence but was over budget. When the hospital launched a huge publicity campaign that focused on its patients receiving respectful, supportive, excellent care, Swedish countered with an advertisement that emphasized high technology and disease treatment. Feedback from doctors was that patients found the Swedish ad more compelling. Although Providence was part of the largest health care system in Washington with its 436 beds, it lost close to $16 million in 1999. At the end of the year the Providence medical director said it was "like a bomb had gone off here."[19]

In 2000, the sisters transferred the acute care hospital and nine remaining clinics to Swedish, which had prospered in the 1990s and was now the largest hospital in the area, with 697 beds. It provided more than $5 million annually to charity care, more than any not-for-profit hospital in the state. Under Swedish ownership, Providence was no longer a Catholic facility. As part of the deal, the Sisters of Providence retained ownership of their hospice, their home care service, and six long-term care facilities. They also obtained more income for their other charity services, including numerous low-income housing projects. Two board members from Providence were added to Swedish's fourteen-member board, and Providence's Sister Susanne Hartung, SP, became director of the new Office of Mission and Ethics at Swedish. Swedish even agreed to Catholic demands to eliminate elective nontherapeutic abortions, although this was amended later.[20]

This was a difficult time in the sisters' health care ministry. Providence Medical Center had served the region for more than 120 years. According to the CEO of the Washington State Medical Association, the transfer reflected the crushing economics and the calamity of the health care delivery system.[21] The president of another hospital warned that the demise of a health care institution that had been around for so long "may represent the loss of a kind of health care tradition and philosophy we won't miss until it's too late."[22]

While the sisters' acute care hospital could not compete with large providers in Seattle, Providence Health System had a better edge in the hospital market in other Washington cities—Everett, Toppenish, and Yakima. In 1994, as the Seattle facility was struggling, Providence Everett merged with Everett General Hospital. The two hospitals had battled for years, notably over which would have a maternity unit in the 1970s and 1980s. Providence leaders in 1978 had agreed to give up the maternity business and when they changed their minds six years later, could not get approved for a certificate of need by the state's Hospital Commission. But Washington's hospitals—including Catholic hospitals—often managed to get around the state's myriad regulations. In 1990, after the Hospital Commission was phased out, Providence set up maternity services that, according to one source, featured oak furniture, views of the mountains, and a Jacuzzi down the hall—difficult for Everett

General to compete with. In 1988 and 1989 both hospitals lost patients, and in 1993 both terminated large numbers of employees and managers. Finally, authorities at Everett General decided to link with Providence to gain access to the large Providence Health System's capital and management depth. The merger put both facilities under the management of the Sisters of Providence, significantly increasing the presence of the Catholic Church in the area; consequently, all abortions and reproductive services other than maternity at the merged institution came to an end.[23]

The sisters in 2003 transferred their hospitals in Yakima and Toppenish, which had generated significant losses, to the for-profit Health Management Associates (HMA), part of a trend of transferring not-for-profit hospitals to for-profit systems that was partly accountable for the expanded role of investor-owned hospitals. The transfer was controversial, but no not-for-profit organization had indicated any interest, while five for-profit agencies had done so. Contract provisions required the net proceeds from the transfer to fund a new community health foundation that would provide ongoing benefits to the local community, to which HMA would contribute $1 million a year.[24]

Providence Health System maintained seventeen other acute care hospitals and twenty long-term care facilities along the West Coast, from Alaska to Southern California, where the Sisters of Providence Health System continued to prosper in the 1990s, with more than $1 billion in revenue.[25]

The example of the Sisters of Providence hospitals in the Northwest reflects not only how hospital integration was successful in some areas and disappointing in others, but also the steps sisters took to maintain their religious ministry. Today, the Sisters of Providence are committed to the frail, low-income elderly. They sponsor Providence Elderplace, which started as a Program of All-Inclusive Care for the Elderly (PACE) demonstration site in 1987. This program integrates Medicare and Medicaid financing in a comprehensive service delivery system. Elderplace has four health and social centers with five hundred enrollees and two residential care facilities with a total of 144 beds attached to the social centers.[26] As the sisters invested in hospice care and facilities for the low-income elderly, they were able to maintain their commitment to respond to unmet needs in the community.

Moving to the Suburbs

In the second half of the twentieth century, partnering with other hospitals to form large systems, as did the Sisters of Providence, was one option for hospitals in an increasingly competitive hospital marketplace. Many other not-for-profit hospitals chose to move from unprofitable inner-city locations serving minority populations to prosperous, primarily white suburbs as sub-urbanization continued to alter the U.S. urban landscape after World War II.[27]

Catholic life before the war included a subculture that had developed in the nineteenth century, as large groups of Irish and German immigrants filled the inner cities in the Northeast and Midwest. Within this subculture were schools, hospitals, and associations of Catholic doctors and lawyers.[28] German Catholic immigrants numbered approximately one and a half million by 1860, and they settled mainly in the German triangle region of Cincinnati, St. Louis, and Milwaukee, which included Chicago.[29]

In 1866, in a heavily German area of Chicago, the historically German Alexian Brothers, under Brother Bonaventure Thelan, CFA, established Alex-ian Brothers Hospital for men and boys. Between 1870 and 1890, the German population of Chicago would triple. The brothers became the hospital's admin-istrators, nurses, x-ray technologists, laboratory technicians, pharmacists, cooks, and physical therapists (see figure 4). As they kept up with modern technology, they constructed four buildings, the last in 1897 on Belden Ave-nue.[30] By 1940, Alexian Brothers Hospital had weathered the Great Depression and was financially stable. It recorded an excess of income over expenses of $11,295, which included deductions from gross earnings of $45,452 in charity care.[31] By the 1950s, the hospital was particularly well known for its care of industrial injuries and of people with alcoholism. It also was the site where most of Chicago's police officers and firefighters received care.[32]

Postwar Chicago experienced massive population shifts as whites moved to northern and western suburbs, among them the wealthier and more socially mobile Catholics. As well, between 1950 and 1979, many private physicians moved from central Chicago to areas with higher socioeconomic status. One study showed a high association between the shifts of doctors' offices and the socioeconomic and racial structure of an area—the postwar suburbs were white enclaves. It was after World War II that inner-city Chicago became a black ghetto.[33]

The experience of the Alexian Brothers Hospital illustrates these demo-graphic changes. In 1959, due to a fall in census at their inner-city hospital, the brothers began considering their hospital's future. The present building was inadequate, with few of the rooms having running water or toilets. An architect counseled building a new structure rather than remodeling. Fac-tors that favored a move out of the city included the makeup of the suburban population—more than 50 percent Catholic—and the shift among German

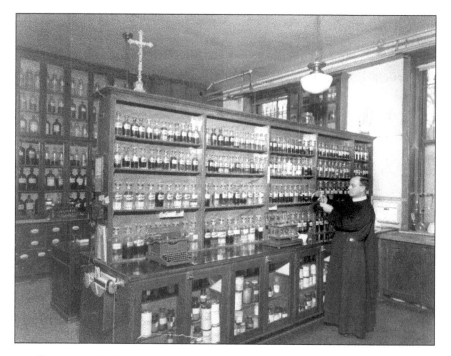

Figure 4   Brother Ludolph Sattler, CFA, in the pharmacy, Chicago, ca. 1945.
Courtesy Alexian Brothers Provincial Archives, Arlington Heights, Illinois.

American Catholics to assimilate into U.S. society, not remain in ethnic enclaves. By 1961 the brothers were discussing moving to a new site; their top choice was Elk Grove, Illinois, the center of the rapidly growing northwest part of the city. The archdiocesan director of hospitals pointed out that industry in the Elk Grove area had increased significantly, which potentially offered the Alexian Brothers more assets for fund-raising. At a Chicago Community Planning meeting in 1961, it was noted of Elk Grove: "If the present population continues to increase, no doubt this area will be a priority in Hill-Burton allocations, in the near future."[34]

On February 21, 1961, the Alexian Brothers Planning Committee recommended building a hospital in Elk Grove Village. They noted that the number of hospitals in the inner city was sufficient to meet the needs of the area, while there was a greater need for a Catholic hospital in the suburbs with their high growth. Land was available and was well located in terms of transportation and housing. And too few physicians used the Alexian Brothers Hospital in the inner city as their first choice. After the brothers obtained all needed permissions, they began plans for construction in 1962. The federal government did indeed recognize the growth potential of the area and allocated $9 million for the new hospital through Hill-Burton funds. In 1963 an auxiliary formed to help raise more money.[35]

The Belden Avenue hospital continued to function, however, and in 1962, after their order's giving six hundred years of health care exclusively to men, the Chicago brothers admitted their first woman patient, a response to doctors' requests and an effort to retain the hospital's solvency.[36] At the same time, the Alexian Brothers worked with a hospital consulting firm and also polled the members of the congregation to determine the fate of the Belden Avenue building once the move took place. One of the consequences of suburbanization was the deterioration of urban neighborhoods, a factor that influenced the Alexian Brothers' decision about the old building. One brother, concerned over the growing secular values in the hospital market, advised that they "destroy the building and sell the property. We are more of a giant corporation than a religious community. . . . If we are to take Vatican II seriously, we must have enough courage to evaluate our vow of poverty." Others did not want to see the property used for something that they themselves could not operate. All agreed that experimentation in new forms of mission work for the congregation should be initiated.[37] In 1968, at the recommendation of the Chicago Hospital Planning Council, the Alexian Brothers decided to close the Belden Avenue hospital, offering compensation packages to employees. In announcing the closing, Brother Flavian Renaud, CFA, provincial of the Immaculate Conception Province, gave three reasons for the painful decision: overabundance of acute care hospitals in the area, inadequate funds to rebuild or repair the existing facility, and lack of brothers to staff two hospitals.[38] In the end, the brothers leased the building as a residence for mentally challenged adults for eight years. They eventually sold it in 1976 to the Little Sisters of the Poor, who had the building demolished later that year in order to build a new nursing home on the site.[39]

Under the administration of Brother Gregory Isenhart, CFA, Saint Alexius Hospital opened in the burgeoning northwestern suburb of Elk Grove Village on June 12, 1966, with 144 beds, 140 on-staff physicians and dentists, and 70 employees. The brothers must have felt that their decision to move had been validated when, in the first month of operation, they serviced 312 patients and 561 emergency clients. In 1971, they renamed the hospital Alexian Brothers Medical Center, as it had expanded to become more than an acute care institution. The four-hundred-bed facility provided care to more than 250,000 patients by 1975, with occupancy rates consistently greater than 80 percent.[40]

In 1971, Alexian Brothers Medical Center initiated a sequence of governance changes that would soon attract national attention. The hospital board of trustees had reorganized, with four laymen and three brothers. The new group changed the medical staff bylaws to state that the hospital's governing board had final responsibility for the quality of care the hospital rendered. This meant that the board would appoint the chief of staff and department chairs; and jointly, with physicians and management, choose physicians (formerly chosen only by the medical staff). In addition, physicians would be answerable to the board through its president rather than directly. These points, the board informed the physicians, were nonnegotiable.[41] The reevaluation of administrative and legal roles was based on two factors. One included rumors that physicians at the hospital were illegally feeding each other business and were keeping poor records, evidence that the doctors were not adequately policing their own. Mainly, however, the decision was based on state and federal legislation, especially the 1965 case *Darling v. Charleston Memorial Hospital*, which involved a malpractice action by an injured football player against a hospital for negligent treatment that resulted in amputation of his leg. In this landmark case in public health legislation, the Illinois Supreme Court established the liability of hospitals, legally and financially, for care provided in their facilities. The ruling held hospitals accountable for protecting patients from unqualified doctors and severely limited physicians' claims of complete authority.[42]

The Alexian Brothers Medical Center board had revised the bylaws without formal adoption by the physicians, and several members of the medical staff attacked both the brothers and the board. The physicians hired a lawyer, and 17 doctors on the 170-member staff resigned. The board countered that it was an accountability issue, and members did not want to rubber stamp medical staff appointments and privileges without investigation.[43] Contending that medical staff bylaws were the prerogative of physicians and that the board's authority was only a ratifying role, angry doctors from Illinois, Arizona, and South Dakota in August 1973 demanded that the American Medical Association House of Delegates condemn the procedure, which it did.[44] Despite the attacks, Alexian Brothers Medical Center eventually added 41 new doctors to its staff, and all agreed to the new bylaws. A drawing factor was a new office building. Standards of the Joint Commission on Accreditation for Hospitals reinforced the Alexian board's decision.[45]

During the 1970s the brothers established a physical rehabilitation unit, psychiatric facility, ambulatory care center, multifaith Department of Religion, Alcoholism Treatment Center, and birthing center. They opened a hospice and home health agency in 1980. The Alexian Brothers of America reorganized in 1983 and created Alexian Brothers Health System, which included, in addition to Elk Grove Village, facilities in Elizabeth, New Jersey; St. Louis, Missouri; San Jose, California; and Signal Mountain, Tennessee.[46]

On April 27, 1980, the brothers held a groundbreaking ceremony for an $8 million expansion project that opened a year later: forty thousand square feet for coronary and intensive care units, new operating rooms, and a nuclear medicine department. In 1984, however, usage dropped significantly in acute care hospitals in the Chicago metropolitan area and surrounding counties, from an occupancy rater of 79.9 percent in 1980 to 69.4 percent in 1984, after the initiation of Diagnostic Related Groups, or DRGs. Furthermore, Illinois's Medicaid contracting program allowed hospitals only a specific number of patients per year at an agreed-upon daily rate, which led to a decrease in Medicaid usage. The Alexian Brothers began expanding into outpatient care, opened primary care services in ambulatory settings, and reached out to Chicago's South Side with a ministry to the Englewood Community. In the mid 1980s they established two off-campus counseling centers, and in 1986 a day hospital treatment center, Samaritan House. They also opened a day surgery unit, sleep lab, and child-care center during this time.[47]

In 1985 the brothers began giving special consideration to the health needs of patients with HIV/AIDS (Human Immunodeficiency Virus/Acquired Immune Deficiency Syndrome). They used their clout as owners of a large medical center to go on record in opposing two Illinois legislature bills that called for mandatory testing and quarantine for HIV/AIDS.[48] They also began planning for a residential facility for these patients, Bonaventure House, and opened it in 1989. At that time, the disease primarily affected gay males, many of whom were professional men who were homeless because they were too sick to work, had been kicked out of their apartments by landlords who feared contracting the disease, or were abandoned by family members because of their lifestyle choices. These factors meshed with the Alexian Brothers ministry to the outsider. It reflected their early work with victims of the Black Death who were abandoned by relatives for becoming sick. Bonaventure House provided room and board, pastoral care, psychosocial counseling, and support groups. This ministry eventually spread to other Illinois cities and to St. Louis, where a similar house became the first Catholic facility for people living with HIV/AIDS in that city and the first dual-diagnosis transitional housing site.[49]

The Alexian Brothers acquired the Northwest Mental Health Center in suburban Chicago in 1997. In a swap with the for-profit Columbia/Hospital Corporation of America (HCA), they announced the acquisition of two facilities, Behavioral Health Hospital and Hoffman Estates Medical Center, in exchange for the brothers' hospital in San Jose, California. The brothers renamed the Hoffman Estates facility Saint Alexius Medical Center. The agreement promised better use of the limited number of brothers in the congregation, and it strengthened their ministries in the Midwest. In 1999, the Health Care Industries Association awarded Saint Alexius Medical Center a 100 Top Hospitals: National Benchmarks for Success award.[50]

The Alexian Brothers balanced market and mission by using the resources of their successful suburban institutions to care for the poor and sick in their HIV/AIDS ministry, which over time increasingly served people with drug addictions.[51] When most health care facilities were questioning their stance on the disease, the Alexian Brothers moved directly into the forefront of care.

A Booming Hospital System

Whereas the Alexian Brothers divested itself of hospitals to concentrate in the Midwest and Northeast, the Daughters of Charity continued to be a national system, and a very successful one at that. Its success can be traced to its parent company, the St. Louis–based Daughters of Charity National Health System (DCNHS), formed in 1986. In 1999, the Daughters joined their health ministry with that of the Sisters of Saint Joseph (of Nazareth) Health System to form Ascension Health, the largest Catholic and largest not-for-profit health system in the country, with hospitals in eighteen states. The DCNHS led the group with nearly eighty hospitals, nursing homes, outpatient clinics, and other health care facilities scattered across fifteen states. One of its most successful networks is the Seton system in Austin, Texas.[52]

Like other congregations, the Daughters of Charity operated many hospitals, orphanages, and educational institutions over the years (see figure 5). After they opened Seton Infirmary in Austin in 1902, they weathered many problems, including influenza and smallpox epidemics in 1916, 1917, and 1918.[53] In 1940, the Daughters changed the name Seton Infirmary to Seton Hospital. They built several additions to the hospital over the years; with a 1953 expansion, the total bed capacity was 225. When the new $1 million wing opened that year, the Daughters offered the general public a tour. A

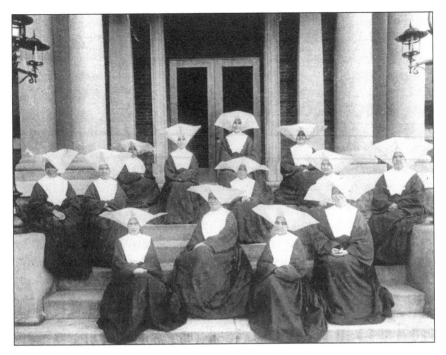

Figure 5   Daughters of Charity of Saint Vincent de Paul, Saint Vincent de Paul Hospital, Birmingham, Alabama, ca. 1906.

Courtesy Barbara Bates Center for the Study of the History of Nursing, University of Pennsylvania, Philadelphia.

prominent feature was the chapel, with two statues reminding people of the Catholic foundation: Saint Vincent de Paul and Saint Louise de Marillac, who established the Daughters of Charity. Eleven nuns comprised the staff, all with bachelor of science degrees in nursing education, along with thirty-eight lay registered nurses. Five of the sisters had completed courses in nursing psychiatry. Others were supervisors with postgraduate degrees.[54]

Seton formed its first lay board of advisors in 1962 and in 1965, after opening their first intensive care unit, the Daughters ran out of land for expansion and began planning to move to a new location in the city. Claude Rainey became the first lay administrator in 1968. The new clinical pharmacy program at the University of Texas began using Seton facilities in 1971. In 1975, when the new hospital facility opened, the board of trustees changed the name to Seton Medical Center. By then, most of Seton's patients came from the middle class and had some type of insurance.[55]

In preparing for a new building, the Daughters could not borrow more than 50 percent, so they obtained financing from Hill-Burton funds, grants by private foundations, the State Department of Health, and a local fund drive.[56] The Seton board of trustees then consisted of seven members of the Daughters of Charity congregation, with trustee committees comprised of both religious and lay people, including Dean Billye Brown of the University of Texas Nursing School. In 1977, fifty-two prominent women of Austin established a Seton Development Board.[57]

Another expansion to the hospital occurred in 1977, and the following year, a regional newborn intensive care unit opened that increased the bed capacity to 450. That same year the Daughters sold the old Seton hospital site for $1.25 million. In 1981, they affiliated with Holy Cross Hospital, formerly operated by the Sisters of Charity of the Incarnate Word, and expanded into East Austin, which serviced a large number of ethnic minorities and the poor. Holy Cross would give the Daughters greater visibility, where they could establish community health, education, and social services. The following year they assumed full responsibility of Holy Cross. In light of federal cutbacks in social programs and rising unemployment, the Daughters were pleased to continue their strong Catholic commitment in East Austin.[58]

With the exception of Claude Rainey's term from 1968 to 1973, Daughters of Charity served as Seton's chief administrators until 1982. By then, Seton had emerged as the leading health care provider in the Austin area, a significant shift from the hospital climate in 1969, when a newspaper article had highlighted the lack of competition among Austin's four hospitals—Holy Cross; Seton; Saint David's Medical Center, originally affiliated with the Episcopal Church and in existence since 1924; and the city-owned Brackenridge. "We should not compete," the had article quoted one administrator, but rather "complement each other." Another stated that hospitals strove to meet community needs rather than meet each other on a competitive basis.[59] By contrast, Seton's *1987 Annual Report* used the language of competition to justify expanding to outlying sites. Saint David's Medical Center had grown into one of the largest health care systems in Texas. Neighboring smaller towns in Central Texas such as Luling also had community hospitals. Differentiating Seton from these institutions could be a key competitive strategy both to prevent other local networks from developing and to give potential patients, managed care plans, and physicians a reason to use Seton rather than other providers. As these neighboring hospitals expanded their bases in Central Texas, they would threaten Seton's market share.[60]

In 1987, Medicare continued to be the leading payer for Seton, at 35.5 percent; Medicare reimbursements at its affiliate, the East Austin landmark, Holy Cross Hospital, totaled 55 percent. Two years later, economic pressures and changing physician referral patterns forced the Daughters of Charity to close Holy Cross. At the same time, they opened the first health center for the working poor in East Austin, Seton East, later renamed McCarthy Community Health Center after Austin bishop John E. McCarthy. In 1988, the Daughters established Seton Northwest Health Plaza in a suburb that had experienced tremendous growth.[61]

The Austin area had a large percentage of poor people, with nearly one out of five in Travis County living below the poverty level. Most used the city-owned Brackenridge Hospital. Seton Medical Center could not serve as a safety net for any but the very poorest and sickest unemployed. In Texas, eligibility for Medicaid was based on federal poverty guidelines, and the state's income threshold to qualify for Medicaid was forty-ninth in the nation—$184 per month for a family of three, compared with the national average of $407 per month. Like other states, Texas reimbursed only a portion of charges under Medicaid. Consequently, in 1991 Seton covered nearly $3.33 million in unpaid Medicaid charges; in two years, Seton's Medicaid losses had increased by 58 percent. Furthermore, during 1991 Seton provided more than $50 million in medical care and other benefits that were uncompensated, a 28 percent increase over the previous year.[62]

In 1995, Seton partnered with Brackenridge Hospital, a move influenced to a great extent by the for-profit Columbia/HCA's entry into the Austin area. Columbia/HCA owned two major hospitals in the city and was in the process of partnering with the new Austin Diagnostic Medical Center and Saint David's Medical Center. By 1998, Seton Medical Center had become a leader in neurology, perinatal nursing, newborn intensive care, eye diseases, and birthing centers. It had specialties in heart disease, cleft lip/palate, urological and gastrointestinal diseases, orthopedics, oncology, and otolaryngology.[63]

Charles Barnett had arrived as CEO in 1993 and had begun developing the Seton Healthcare Network. A native of Ohio, Barnett held bachelor's and master's degrees in the history of medicine and a master's degree in hospital administration. Starting off as an operating room technician, he had a long history of work in many hospital departments, which gave him an understanding of hospitals from the ground up that proved a distinct advantage. By the late 1990s, Seton Healthcare Network was the third largest private employer in the region, with six thousand employees. In 1996 it opened Seton

South, a second community health center serving the working poor. Seton Cove, a spirituality center, became part of the network the next year.[64] The financially strapped Edgar B. Davis Memorial Hospital in the rural area of Luling had recently transferred to Seton and expected the large network to get it back on its feet financially, according to one Luling City Council member: "They've got deeper pockets than we do, and if anyone's going to keep our hospital open, they're going to do it." As other facilities joined the Seton Healthcare Network, it became the largest regional health center in the area, with gross revenues in 1998 of $729 million, up 16.8 percent from the previous year.[65]

As it branched into new services and towns, Seton was fast becoming what one newspaper article labeled the "800 pound gorilla of health care in Central Texas."[66] Many of the new programs gave clients greater access to health care—home care services, a teen parenting center, and an emergency relief endowment.[67] By 2008, Seton Family of Hospitals included facilities in six counties; it was the leading provider of health care services in Central Texas. Its total operating revenue was $1.25 billion, with labor costs of $545 million and other operating expenses of $607 million. Seton's charity care totaled $285 million, by far the most of any hospital system in the region. Reinvestments to meet community needs included $210 million for technology, infrastructure, and construction of new facilities. The Seton Health Plan provided insurance to 14,500 Central Texans, and it remains the largest Children's Health Insurance Program (CHIP) provider in the Travis County service area.[68]

This rapid growth can be attributed to several factors. In January 1998, when the *Wall Street Journal* referred to the Daughters of Charity as "the Daughters of Currency," analysts noted that "key Daughters' hospitals are located not in inner-city areas but in more affluent suburbs." According to the article, the DCNHS received 60 percent of its income from investments, compared with a "fifty-fifty split of profits between hospitals and investments." Like other not-for-profit hospitals, the Daughters used their profits for charitable purposes. But because they held the reserves for the benefit of the hospitals, the investment income was not taxed, and it grew. A Seton spokesperson noted that the $2 billion investment fund gave the Daughters a "strong financial base to weather changes in a volatile environment," but there was no "purposeful strategy to grow reserves and sit on them." According to the Daughters of Charity, their success resulted from their careful stewardship of resources. By 1998, the DCNHS's largest savings came from divesting the network of eleven unprofitable hospitals.[69] In addition, not only did the Daughters hire experienced CEOs such as Charles Barnett, but also they developed a board of trustees whose members worked in information technology, academic nursing schools, architecture, and financial services.

Indicating the persistent tension between market and mission, the editor of a Catholic publication noted: "Hospitals can hardly care for paying patients let alone the poor if they are bleeding red ink."[70]As Sister Irene Kraus, DC, head of the DCNHS, told the *Wall Street Journal*: "No market, no mission."[71] In taking this tough stance, the Daughters consistently emphasized charity as their main goal. Their expansion in Austin helped them meet community needs by making them even more accessible to Central Texans, who had historically come to Seton's facilities.

History of a Transfer

The Sisters of Mercy hospital in Pittsburgh experienced a different trajectory. Founded in 1847, Mercy Hospital adapted its services to the continuing shifts in demand of its urban populace. For example, as the steel and coal industries grew in the late nineteenth and early twentieth centuries, the hospital became a treatment center for industrial injuries. By the early twentieth century, it had expanded to 670 beds, aided by donors such as the Frick family. During the Great Depression the hospital's bed usage dropped, but the Hospital Council of Allegheny County's adoption of Blue Cross in 1937 led to a rise in occupancy rates. Blue Cross went into effect January 1, 1938, and that year Mercy adopted the Group Hospitalization Plan. "From an economic point of view the service has added nothing to the income of the hospital," noted Mercy's *1939 Annual Report*, "but neither has it been a liability"; the hospital had an occupancy rate of 83 percent and admitted 12,599 patients. In 1940, it admitted the largest number of patients in its history, 13,866, with an 88 percent occupancy rate. Hospitalization insurance covered 43 percent of patients in 1944.[72]

In the first half of the twentieth century, Mercy Hospital was one of the foremost hospitals in western Pennsylvania. Well-known specialists in surgery and medicine treated its trauma and cancer patients. It offered residencies in many different specialties and was known for its pioneer anesthesiology department. Its position at the pinnacle declined during the 1950s, mainly as a result of the University of Pittsburgh medical school, which preferred to train its students in its own facilities; its 1950s expansion reduced the number of medical students Mercy physicians taught. The University of Pittsburgh also attracted full-time doctors such as Jonas Salk, whose team's research led to the development of the first polio vaccine. With full-time teaching faculty at the university, Mercy's physicians as part-time lecturers there became less important to the teaching program. To expand Mercy's teaching role and make its internships and residencies more marketable, under the direction of Sister Carlotta Vanvoy, RSM, the hospital in 1951 raised its room rates; this allowed it to pay interns $100 and residents $150 per month.[73]

Mercy Hospital was situated in the heart of the city, a location that was central to renovation efforts that later became known as the Pittsburgh Renaissance, the Smoky City's postwar urban renewal project that included cleaning up its rivers, controlling air pollution, and constructing new buildings. The years 1953 to 1978, under the administration of Sister Ferdinand Clark, RSM, were pivotal to Mercy's growth and expansion.[74] Sister Ferdinand held teaching certificates from the State of Pennsylvania and the Diocese of Pittsburgh; she had taught in an elementary school and served as admissions officer at Mercy Hospital and as the superior at Saint Paul's Orphanage. In 1956 Duquesne University made her an honorary doctor of education.[75]

When Sister Ferdinand took over Mercy's administration in 1953, she inherited a 688-bed hospital with an annual admission of eighteen thousand, many of whom received free care. An outpatient clinic treated nearly twenty-three thousand patients at no charge. In addition to the presence of fifty Sisters of Mercy, the hospital employed a thousand people and had a hundred physicians on staff. With donations from Pittsburgh residents, Sister Ferdinand and a new cadre of physicians supervised the upgrading of deteriorating buildings, added new specialties such as nuclear medicine (1954), expanded the Social Service Department, established a regional burn unit (1967), required an increase in medical research, and enhanced teaching opportunities for medical students, interns, and residents. In 1962, as white middle-class residents moved to the suburbs, hospital consultant Eugene Rosenfeld recommended that Mercy Hospital stay in the city.[76] A suburban location would have benefited both the sisters and the new community, but it would have hurt the poor; the sisters decided to stay.

The early administration at Mercy Hospital differed from that of other U.S. Catholic hospitals. In the late nineteenth and early twentieth centuries, a lay board of trustees administered its affairs; not until 1913 was a sister elected to the board. Between 1923 and 1947, however, sisters gradually replaced all lay members, although a lay advisory board was formed in 1952 as a liaison between the hospital and the city. In 1964, the Mercy board of trustees once again became primarily a lay board, comprised of six sisters and thirty leaders of elite Pittsburgh businesses (see figure 6). This board composition did not accord with the rules and regulations of the Catholic Church and the Catholic Hospital Association (CHA), and many of the sisters themselves feared a loss of autonomy. Once the CHA and the Sisters of Mercy were convinced that the board would handle management affairs and fund-raising while the sisters maintained ownership of the hospital, however, they approved the board makeup. Yet this move took away the sisters' right to appoint the board, approve the president, and approve changes to the bylaws. Although the first layman in hospital administration was hired in 1965 as assistant administrator, a Sister of Mercy continued to hold the highest administrative position until 1998.[77]

In the 1960s, the idea of relocation to the suburbs persisted, and in 1971 the topic of moving again arose when Mercy leaders began planning for a new six-hundred-bed hospital expansion. The Hospital Planning Association

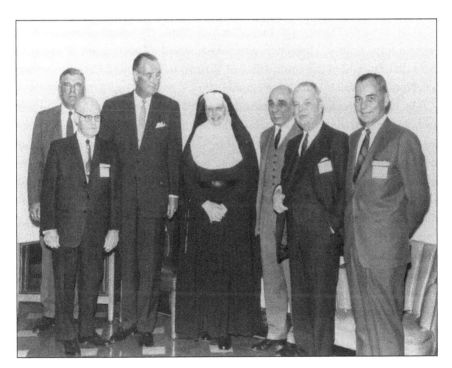

Figure 6   Sister Ferdinand Clark, RSM, with Mercy Hospital Board of Trustees, Pittsburgh, ca. 1964.

Courtesy Archives, UPMC Mercy, Pittsburgh, Pennsylvania.

(HPA), developed to control spiraling hospital costs and consisting of corporate leaders in the city, was responsible for approving any major hospital
expansion in the area. In the 1960s the HPA had turned down Mercy's request
for renovations without a more thorough evaluation of the hospital and hinted
that Mercy should move to the suburbs.[78]

But in 1971 the HPA approved the expansion project based on the submission of a long-range plan that outlined Mercy's role as a major teaching institution and specialty hospital. Mercy Health Center, the outpatient care facility,
had developed to serve the needs of the surrounding indigent community.[79] It
was not lost on hospital planners that a move to the suburbs would threaten
Mercy's role as a teaching hospital, partly because, as one report noted, in the
city Mercy was surrounded by a high incidence of diseases peculiar to low-
income areas, such as chronic lung diseases, tuberculosis, venereal disease,
and malnutrition, which would not be found in suburbia. Again the sisters
decided not to move. With HPA approval, they undertook the construction of
a thirteen-story tower in 1973, aided by nearly $6 million from benefactors
such as U.S. Steel, Gulf Oil, the Mellon Foundation, and Westinghouse Elec-
tric Corporation. Throughout the 1970s and 1980s, the hospital continued to
receive large grants. The sisters also inaugurated a Department of Pastoral
Care that, in light of the ecumenism of Vatican II, included a Catholic priest,
a Protestant chaplain, and a Jewish rabbi.[80]

In 1978, Sister Joanne Marie Andiorio, RSM, succeeded Sister Ferdinand
as executive director of Mercy Hospital. She was a graduate of Carlow College, where she had served as a reference librarian. Her tenure coincided
with the decline of Pittsburgh's reign as the center of the steel industry. As
unemployment rates soared, the city reinvented itself on the basis of new
service and health care fields and high-tech industries. In 1983, Mercy Hospital reorganized into the Pittsburgh Mercy Health System (PMHS), a holding
company that included Mercy Hospital and Mercy Hospital Foundation. This
reorganization strengthened the Sisters of Mercy sponsorship by returning
to them the right to approve the president and changes to the corporation's
bylaws, which they had lost in 1964 to the lay board of trustees (why lay
board members were willing to cede power back to the sisters is unexplained
by the available material). The reorganization also protected Mercy's funds
in a way that allowed the hospital to stay in the inner city and provide several million dollars of free care. New buildings constructed then included
cardiovascular and maternity centers, a neonatal intensive care unit, and an
emergency trauma center.[81] In 1985, Mercy's corporate structure changed yet

again: the sisters agreed to participate in the Eastern Mercy Health System, sponsored by Sisters of Mercy from Maine to Florida.

By the 1990s, all Pittsburgh hospitals were exploring linkages to eliminate duplication of services and lower health care costs. Pittsburgh Mercy Health System purchased Saint John's Hospital in 1989 and Divine Providence Hospital in 1993. Over time, PMHS included Mercy Jeannette Hospital, Mercy Behavioral Health (originally part of Saint John's Hospital), and Mercy Senior Care, along with several primary care and outpatient treatment centers.[82] Mercy Hospital of Pittsburgh remained in the black in 1990, with Medicare paying 51.6 percent of charges, Blue Cross 22.6 percent, and Medicaid 10 percent. In contrast, and in line with other hospitals experiencing financial difficulties, Mercy Psychiatric Institute's finances relied on Medicaid for more than half its charges, Medicare for 22.9 percent, and Blue Cross for only 8.9 percent. Hospitals that brought in relatively more money from patients covered with commercial insurance were more successful than hospitals that relied more on Medicaid reimbursements.[83] In 1993, while Mercy Hospital of Pittsburgh had a net income of over $3 million, Mercy Providence Hospital and other acquisitions such as Mercy Center for Chemical Dependency Services suffered financial losses.[84]

"Chaos" was the word that best described the health care situation in western Pennsylvania, according to a writer for the *Pittsburgh Business Times* in May 1996.[85] As hospital occupancy levels dropped to 61 percent, leaders desperately sought closer relationships, mergers, and acquisitions. The University of Pittsburgh Medical Center (UPMC) went on a buying spree, announcing its willingness to spend $300 million to achieve a presence in all markets of the state.[86] To improve their revenue base, Pittsburgh Mercy Health System and the Western Pennsylvania Healthcare System partnered with 150 primary care physicians in a for-profit physician-run group, but the venture fell through in 1997. West Penn wanted to merge with PMHS; PMHS was not interested.[87] Yet PMHS was experiencing slowing revenue growth, attributable in part to the federal Balanced Budget Act of 1997, and in part to the need to integrate the many hospitals it had already acquired.[88]

Adding to the chaos was the demise of the Allegheny Health Education and Research Foundation (AHERF) in 1998. In the 1990s, Pittsburgh's Allegheny General Hospital, part of AHERF, was UPMC's chief rival. As reimbursements from third-party payers shrank, AHERF had rapidly expanded into Pittsburgh and Philadelphia, acquiring hospitals, physicians, and medical schools. In light of its increased debt and large cash transfers, AHERF eventually had to file for bankruptcy—the largest not-for-profit health care failure in the country.[89] The same year, Eastern Mercy Health System had joined with the Sisters of Providence and the non-Catholic Allegheny Health Systems to form Catholic Health East. When AHERF's flagship hospital, Allegheny General, had to find a buyer, the likely candidate was Catholic Health East, now the parent company of Pittsburgh Mercy Health System. When Western Pennsylvania Hospital System also made a bid for Allegheny General, Catholic Health East dropped out of the bidding, and Allegheny General and other hospitals transferred to the smaller West Penn system in 1999.[90]

The region would witness the impact of other closures. Saint Francis Health System, Pittsburgh's only other Catholic health group, closed its facilities in 2001, with huge social consequences for Mercy. Saint Francis had been recognized for its psychiatric programs and alcohol addiction services, and Mercy absorbed this patient population, many of whom could not pay and had no health insurance.[91] In 2007, after losing money for several years, Pittsburgh Mercy Health System refocused its mission and transferred its acute care services to other providers in the region, with a resulting loss of control over Mercy Hospital of Pittsburgh, which the Sisters of Mercy had owned for more than 150 years. In January 2008, Mercy Hospital merged with the University of Pittsburgh Medical Center. As the president of the Pittsburgh Sisters of Mercy stated: "I did not want to have another St. Francis"—that is, she did not want to see Mercy shut down altogether.[92]

This was a strategic move. Under the University of Pittsburgh Medical Center, Mercy Hospital of Pittsburgh would remain Catholic, thereby ensuring a Catholic presence in the community. Remaining part of PMHS were a parish nursing program; Mercy Behavioral Health; Operation Safety Net, a program for the homeless; and A Child's Place, for children suspected of being abused. According to the Pittsburgh Mercy Health System Web site, the Sisters of Mercy "returned to their roots of caring for the most vulnerable people in the community. . . . Today, PMHS provides services to the most at-risk residents of the community—those facing mental illness, addictions, homelessness, abuse, and isolation."[93]

At the end of the twentieth century, the University of Pittsburgh Medical Center retained its prominence and prestige. It had established a competitive advantage over Mercy Hospital in the 1950s when researchers such as Salk were hired, and the medical center could offer superior research and medical education. While it expanded in the 1990s, Pittsburgh Mercy Health System hospitals' debts increased. Even though Mercy Hospital of Pittsburgh had been successful financially, the other less-well-off hospitals vied for the system's pooled capital, which drained the stronger institution. The sisters' transfer of Mercy Hospital of Pittsburgh to UPMC helped the nuns preserve their charitable mission, and proceeds of the transaction were used to form McAuley Ministries, a public foundation and the grant-making arm of what remained of Pittsburgh Mercy Health System.

Going It Alone: A Safety-Net Hospital

The intensifying competition among hospitals in the last quarter of the twentieth century drove increased demand for safety-net hospitals, institutions widely recognized in the community as serving low-income and uninsured people. Mercy Hospital and Medical Center in Chicago, owned and operated by the Sisters of Mercy, is considered such an institution. Between 1996 and 2005, a Community Tracking Study reported that the number of uninsured people nationally had increased by 13 percent. While American Hospital Association data showed that uncompensated care costs increased by 28 percent in the 1990s, they had decreased as a percentage of total hospital expenses by 7 percent, partly because private practice physicians had decreased the amount of charity care they provided. The effect on safety-net hospitals was a rising demand for services among the uninsured and Medicaid patients.[94]

The first Catholic hospital established in Chicago, Mercy Hospital and Medical Center, has had a presence there since 1851. In the early years, the sisters received criticism for not admitting blacks to their acute care hospital. In 1921, however, the Sisters of Mercy took over the management of the Mercy Free Dispensary, which offered free basic care to neighborhood residents, many of whom were black. That year, a Mercy Hospital fund-raising advertisement compared the hospital to a long-running piece of machinery: "Business men would give millions for a machine that would run 27,394 days without stopping. The Sisters of Mercy have served the city of Chicago for 27,394 days up to September 25, 1921." They had cared for the sick and orphans, educated children and adults, "relieved the poor, and comforted the unfortunate. No machine devised by man could do any of these things."[95]

Dispensaries served as training institutions for medical students, such as those from Loyola University. Mercy physicians and students staffed Mercy Free Dispensary, which depended on the hospital for financial, laboratory, x-ray, and pharmacy support, with money from the government, Loyola University, the local community fund, and donations.[96] The dispensary was an important outpatient ministry for the sisters, but financing it was not easy. In 1932, the hospital superior wrote to Father Ahearn at Loyola University: "Mercy Dispensary belongs to Mercy Hospital and the Hospital is willing for the School of Medicine to use the dispensary for teaching purposes. For the dispensary to be effective as a teaching unit there must of necessity be a number of free beds available" in the hospital, for which the Medical School should bear the cost. For years, she wrote, Mercy Hospital had carried the burden of expenses, while "the Medical School has seemingly been unconcerned," but Mercy could no longer do that. The sisters were willing to provide x-ray and electrocardiograph machines, but the Medical School would have to cover expenses for patients too poor to pay. In 1935, the sisters closed the dispensary due to financial problems, then reopened it in 1938.[97] Over the next decades, under the sisters' management, financing the dispensary remained problematic. In 1952, they opened a Home Medical Care Program for patients unable to come to the dispensary; in 1953, they had to cover the dispensary's deficit of $26,000. Ten years later, it ranked as one of the busiest clinics in the city.[98]

In 1954, the Sisters of Mercy agreed to move from Chicago's Near South Side, a primarily working-class and poor section of the city, to Skokie, Illinois, in the more affluent North Side, with Loyola University Medical School, which had been renamed the Stritch School of Medicine. Mercy's South Side neighborhood had deteriorated as industries and small businesses moved away, and robberies and attacks on nurses and other personnel were common. But tensions between the sisters and Stritch School of Medicine at Loyola over questions of independence and control simmered for five years. The Stritch dean saw the School of Medicine running the hospital as a laboratory for its students, while the sisters wanted to maintain an independent hospital to serve the sick. As Mother Mary Regina Cunningham, RSM, provincial of the Sisters of Mercy in Chicago, noted in 1961: "Control of the hospital must rest with the Sisters. Control of the students and their instruction rests with the Medical School." The disagreement culminated in the sisters' deciding to stay and build a new building at their Near South Side location.[99]

Most important, local physicians and South Siders wanted the sisters to remain there. Mercy's outpatient clinic had sixty thousand annual visits, far more than would be the case in the more financially stable Skokie. Thus by the 1960s, Mercy Hospital was pursuing an independent course. In 1969 a new Stritch School of Medicine and 504-bed teaching hospital opened at Loyola University Medical Center in Maywood, Illinois. Mercy was not affiliated with any one medical school for several years but eventually established teaching affiliations with Loyola and the University of Illinois College of Medicine.[100]

In the 1960s and 1970s, an urban renewal project helped clean up the area surrounding Mercy Hospital. Michael Reese Hospital and the Illinois Institute of Technology expanded their facilities in the South Side, and new middle-class housing units opened. This growth influenced Mercy's decision to remain in place, and new buildings were constructed in 1968 and 1976. Three Chicago business and civic leaders were elected in 1972 as the first lay people on the hospital's board of directors, a policy-making and voting group. The sisters maintained control, however, as the other ten members of the board were all Sisters of Mercy.[101]

Chicago's inner city remained one of the nation's most segregated areas, and Mercy's outpatient clinic continued to have a large number of patient visits. In the 1970s, the clinic became the Harry and Maribel Blum Diagnostic and Treatment Center and expanded its services to thirty specialties. Sisters also established a Community Guidance Center for outpatient psychological services, an Alcoholic and Drug Treatment Unit, and a Children's Learning Disabilities Center. The emergency room became known for its care of trauma patients. In 1976 the hospital changed its official name to Mercy Hospital and Medical Center.[102]

Mercy's *1981 Annual Report* revealed that revenues exceeded expenses by $22 million, a 2.8 percent return, according to administrator Sister Sheila Lyne, RSM, which was average for the hospital industry and "excellent for a hospital whose patient days are accounted for by 21 percent Medicaid; 36 percent Medicare; 19 percent commercial insurance coverage; 15 percent Blue Cross; 4 percent self paid; and 5 percent uncollectibles." By 1985 Mercy had a 72 percent occupancy rate, significantly above the 66 percent average for other Chicago hospitals. Mercy had responded to changing hospital utilization through services that reflected increased consumer usage, such as a home health care program, Mercy Healthcare and Rehabilitation Center, and an immediate care center.[103]

The Chicago-area hospitals illustrate the influence of the Catholic hierarchy on hospital affiliations. In 1986 Chicago's Joseph Cardinal Bernardin proposed a Catholic Health Alliance that would join all twenty-three of the city's powerful but financially suffering Catholic hospitals. No other health care provider came close to matching their collective presence in the city; their more than four thousand beds accounted for more than one-fourth of the city's total. In addition, Sister Sheila, who had become the city's health commissioner, held a powerful leadership position, the first woman in that post.[104] Bernardin saw that if the hospitals linked their assets, cut costs, curtailed ineffective services, and closed marginal institutions, the resulting alliance would be a remarkable player in the city's hospital marketplace. What made the proposed association precarious was the concern over who would control it, the Chicago Archdiocese or the individual religious congregations that owned and operated the hospitals. Catholic hospitals competed not only with non-Catholic institutions but also among themselves.

The Catholic Health Alliance was not due to materialize for some time, and in 1994, as Chicago's hospitals entered into a frenzy of consolidations, Bernardin threatened to withdraw the Catholic status of any hospital in his archdiocese that refused to join the Catholic network.[105] The threat was not carried out. In 1995, while being treated for pancreatic cancer, the cardinal wrote "A Sign of Hope: A Pastoral Letter on Healthcare," expressing his concern that health care was being viewed primarily as a business commodity, a position that Catholic hospitals should counter. One of his basic convictions was the idea of "being there": "Illness is a kind of human exile. . . . We must recognize the absolute necessity of being present as a community to others in need." In his mind, Catholic hospitals did this better than any others.[106]

To be there for patients, however, required a stable financial picture, and competitive pressures had eroded Mercy Hospital and Medical Center's financial record, which scared away potential affiliates. If it was to survive, noted one leader, the hospital had to be both business oriented and faith based.[107] Throughout the mid and late twentieth century, Mercy had benefited from the philanthropy of politicians such as former U.S. representative Dan Rostenkowski and the Catholic mayor Richard J. Daley, who both had family members still involved in advisory boards and fund-raisers. But in 1999, the hospital was serving a neighborhood of mostly low- to moderate-income residents, and 60 percent of its admissions relied on Medicare and Medicaid, which continued to have low reimbursement rates. As safety-net providers such as Mercy absorbed these funding shortfalls, they also were providing more uncompensated care. To complicate the picture, Mercy lost $39 million in the fiscal year ending June 30, 2000, through a series of management mistakes by lay executives over the previous two years.[108]

Among the problems Catholic sisters across the country faced at the turn of the twenty-first century was their loss of control over management operations. A board of trustees had been established in the 1960s to give policy oversight, and although the Sisters of Mercy continued to hold controlling sponsorship of the Chicago hospital, the sisters on the board in 2000 felt duped by the managers who had kept them in the dark about the hospital's financial problems over the preceding years. Sister Lenore Mulvihill, RSM, chair of the board, reported: "We weren't being told the truth. I was awake nights . . . knowing this hospital had been [here] for 150 years and now this was happening under my watch and the watch of the Board." She and the other board members brought in consultants from national firms to assist them and rehired Sister Sheila, who left her job as the city's health officer to take over as CEO of Mercy.[109]

With a master's degree in psychiatric nursing from Saint Xavier and an MBA from the University of Chicago, Sister Sheila had been chief executive at the hospital from 1976 to 1991. In a 2009 interview with me, she spoke about the shift of health care from "the public good to a marketable commodity": "I try to throw this expression out every now and then," she said. "I'm concerned that the reaction generally, although it's not spoken, [is] . . . 'There she goes again.' Another thing they could be saying is, 'She doesn't get it; this is a big business.' And you know, in terms of money and financing, . . . I'll give you that, but what are you using all of that for? Was it ever intended to make a million and a half as a CEO? As a public good and to make it a marketable commodity to justify it? I just see too much of that in Illinois."[110]

Mercy Hospital and Medical Center continued to experience financial pressures. One of its sources of income was a provider tax levied on the city's hospitals, to which the federal government added, and from which hospitals received a percentage back. The aim was to redistribute more of the money to safety-net hospitals, but these institutions had to compete with large medical centers that also serviced Medicaid patients such as Northwestern, which got a significant percentage of the provider tax.[111]

To increase revenue, Mercy Hospital leaders focused on attracting more privately insured patients, more federal dollars, private contributions, and state funds. Broader specialty services included a Heart and Vascular Care Center and a Comprehensive Breast Care Center. The Harry and Maribel Blum Diagnostic and Treatment Center became a federally qualified health center, a benefit under Medicare for safety-net hospitals to enhance the provision of primary care services in underserved urban and rural areas. By 2002, Mercy's private contributions had increased by 25 percent. Mayor Richard M. Daley, who was born at Mercy, and Governor George Ryan were supportive, and other state politicians secured $4.5 million in public funds. As an essential element of Mercy's fulfillment of its mission, Sister Sheila established a Spiritual Care and Patient Advocacy Center, where counselors offered one-on-one counseling and bereavement support to patients, family members, and staff.[112] She and a priest in pastoral services started meeting personally with departments to go over mission values. She said: "We try real hard to make them feel good about themselves. We do spend time with that."[113]

But Mercy's financial status remained tenuous, and Sister Sheila eliminated extra benefits for the management and nursing staff. Bondholders pushed Mercy leaders to sell or merge with a larger player to bring in cash, which would pay off bondholders while ensuring that the hospital stayed open. Mercy did seek partnerships, and several hospitals considered alliances, among them a for-profit hospital, the likes of which Cardinal Bernardin had criticized in the 1990s. His successor, Francis Cardinal George, supported Bernardin's stance and continued to work with the sisters to find a not-for-profit buyer or partner. By then, however, no one wanted to align with the financially strapped hospital. In the meantime, the sisters sold to developers land that was located close to the acute care facility, and the hospital hoped to benefit by a gentrification of the surrounding neighborhood.[114]

By 2008, under Sister Sheila, the institution had developed nationally recognized heart and cancer programs. She also headed a $24 million capital improvement plan. The hospital expanded its presence in the local community by investing money in vocational career training programs and national youth leadership forums on medicine.[115] Mercy Hospital and Medical Center remained a stand-alone facility, however. It shared resources such as payroll, personnel, and rehabilitation services with Saint Bernard's and Saint Anthony's, other Catholic stand-alone hospitals in the area.[116]

As leaders at Mercy Hospital and Medical Center chose to stay in the Near South Side, they found that maintaining the balance between mission and financial viability was especially problematic for a safety-net hospital. The hospital weathered the threats by increasing its recognition in the community as a provider of specialty care and by attracting more paying, middle-class patients. Yet, close to 40 percent of its revenue still comes from Medicaid, nearly three times the national average of 14 percent.[117] As it continues to provide care for the poor as a stand-alone facility, the probability that it will suffer financially increases.

Conclusion

Throughout their history, Catholic sisters and brothers in the health care field have adapted to the U.S. hospital market. In the twentieth century, they prepared themselves spiritually and professionally, many earning advanced degrees. Following the trend in higher education, most congregations moved their schools of nursing into collegiate programs. During the Great Depression,

Catholic hospitals turned to Blue Cross insurance for solutions to their financial problems. And after Vatican II, sisters and brothers had new insights into collegiality and working with the laity. For all Catholic hospitals, however, the years after Vatican II and the instigation of Medicare and Medicaid were indeed precarious ones. As James C. Robinson has argued, health care leaders had to adapt to the vagaries of reimbursements. Hospitals moved away from providing only acute care services into a variety of areas where reimbursement was more favorable. They developed ambulatory care centers, chronic care facilities, and specialty hospitals.[118] Lease agreements, mergers, and acquisitions between Catholic and secular hospitals increased, creating hybrid religious and secular institutions that demonstrated unprecedented flexibility for Catholic sisters and brothers as sponsors of hospitals.

In the 1960s all hospitals benefited from increased government payments through Medicare and Medicaid, which paid for many patients previously served as charity cases. Both programs were primary sources of revenue, with Medicaid paying the safety-net hospitals and others that served a disproportionate share of the uninsured. Medicaid also increased access to needed services for the poor. But by itself, Medicaid did not go far enough to eliminate disparities among hospitals. As the uninsured population grew, people more often used local emergency departments for acute care services, which contributed to uncompensated hospital expenses. In addition, Medicare and Medicaid had disadvantages: as government regulation of their financial and operational sides grew, hospitals lost autonomy.[119]

At the same time, many Catholic religious congregations were among the most successful service providers in the country for a number of reasons. As hospital bureaucracies grew, sisters and brothers hired CEOs or assistant CEOs, either lay or religious, with MBAs. With skills in managing large institutions already in place, many sisters and brothers adapted easily to the large corporate systems formed in the 1980s and 1990s, which helped Catholic hospitals maintain their identity and commitment to each other. Multihospital systems increased Catholic influence in the secular marketplace through providing a strong base to promote Catholic philosophy, beliefs, and attitudes on healing as a ministry and on the value of human dignity. Indeed, Catholic systems preserved the plurality of the hospital marketplace and ensured a strong Catholic presence.[120]

Each religious congregation responded as it had to in order to survive. Many could look at the larger picture to identify assets and potential problems, services that would attract physicians, and technology and other resources needed to obtain paying patients. They began developing the financially lucrative service of cardiovascular care. The Daughters of Charity and the Alexian Brothers thrived with their key hospitals located in primarily middle-class areas, and the Daughters especially were adamant about keeping a sizeable financial reserve. As many of the Catholic systems, like other not-for-profit and for-profit systems, found themselves part of large "overbuilt organizations," some congregations were willing to divest themselves of some hospitals to increase their strength with others.[121]

Leaders at Mercy Hospital in Chicago made different choices and continued to struggle with their safety-net hospital close to the inner city. To increase the number of paying patients, they eventually added cardiovascular services and cancer programs. Although the hope was that multihospital systems could provide supportive services to the weaker hospitals in the group, this was not always the case. Mercy Hospital of Pittsburgh's support of the financially struggling institutions in its system was not enough. As Pittsburgh Mercy Health System expanded rapidly in the 1990s, it accumulated substantial debts, provided large amounts of charity care, and eventually transferred ownership to another hospital system. At the same time, the Pittsburgh Sisters of Mercy were able to preserve their charitable mission by launching into new service areas.

Over the twentieth century, Catholic hospital leaders had to make difficult choices to maintain economic sustainability as they struggled to compete in the secular medical marketplace. At the same time, for all Catholic sisters and brothers still in health care, a refocus from acute care hospitals to social services such as HIV/AIDs care, hospice, and home health care, areas neglected by current funding, was a way for them to meet needs of the poor and elderly.[122]

Chapter 3

Religion, Gender, and the Public Representation of Catholic Hospitals

"Experiencing the physical dimension of religion," Colleen McDannell has noted, "helps bring about religious values, norms, behaviors, and attitudes."[1] As Catholic hospitals partnered with non-Catholic facilities in the late twentieth century, they faced challenges in their religious identities. This was not the case in the century's earlier decades. During that era, patients could experience the divine through both the religious women and men who attended them and the religious images and symbols that surrounded them. This was one of the ways that Catholic sisters and brothers distinguished themselves and their hospitals from secular facilities. They conceived of illness not only in biological terms but also within a spiritual framework, and they viewed themselves as spiritual agents of care. Catholic hospitals were places where people could obtain not only physical healing but also a "good death." These tangible signs, symbols, and beliefs informed Catholics who they were and identified their institutions to non-Catholics.[2] Sisters and brothers used written sources as well as unwritten texts—images of buildings, clothing, art, and photographs—to market their religious messages to their patients and to the general public. A visitor to a Catholic hospital in the early twentieth century saw fonts of holy water and paintings of the bishop, the Virgin Mary, and saints. These places powerfully influenced the meaning of nursing for the women, men, and nursing students who worked in them.

Analyses of nursing have paid attention to representations, mainly of women, through photographs and writings. Representation involves how people and institutions present themselves to the public through paintings, symbols, stories, photographs, written communications, and practices. Although such sources do not indicate actual lived experiences, they can be useful for investigating the role of religion and gender in constituting social interactions.[3] Over the course of the twentieth century, religious and gendered representations changed as Catholic beliefs and practices changed; nevertheless, religion persisted with relation to Catholic hospitals, albeit in different ways.

Public Representations of Religion: The U.S. Catholic Hospital

In the first half of the twentieth century, Catholic leaders marketed their health care institutions as including "sacred" space within the "medical" space of the hospital. Hospital art and architecture were important in the visual projection of a sacred Catholic identity. Catholicism's acceptance of paintings, sculptures, and other religious icons distinguished it from the Protestant tradition, which shunned icons and emphasized preaching. To Catholics, however, artworks were signs that mediated religious meanings. Sisters and brothers held processionals in their hospitals, accompanied patients to masses in hospital chapels, and held devotions to the saints to remind patients of their faith. These practices conveyed a distinct religious vision and were important in a religion such as Catholicism that emphasized ritual.[4]

In the nineteenth to the mid-twentieth century, devotions were very much a part of Catholic spirituality. As McDannell asserts: "Catholics learned and accepted the reality of a supernatural community because they were taught how to interact with it through their devotional practices."[5] In the nineteenth century the Catholic Church had revived exercises such as the rosary, forty hours' devotion, benediction, and devotions to the Sacred Heart and the Immaculate Conception. Devotions to the saints and the Virgin Mary, who, Catholics believed, had power over disease, were especially important. Devotions were a form of popular religion that acted as a bridge between the intellectual teachings of the Church and the expression of one's personal piety. They could help concretize certain tenets of Catholicism, such as redemption. For example, veneration of the Blessed Sacrament reflected the Catholic doctrine of the real presence of Christ. Novenas, or nine-day devotions, honored a saint or supported a particular request. Relics were popular, and sisters and brothers used beads, scapulars, medals, and holy pictures to lead a patient closer to God. Religious clothing, another physical representation of religion, could mark a boundary between a sister or brother and members of the laity.[6] Catholic hospitals' religious buildings, architecture, art, clothing, use of devotions, and other specific practices were created by Catholic

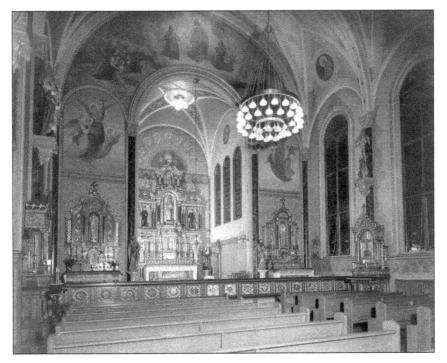

Figure 7   Chapel, Alexian Brothers Hospital, Chicago, ca. 1937.
Courtesy Alexian Brothers Provincial Archives, Arlington Heights, Illinois.

brothers and sisters to provide a world of religious meaning for their patients
and nursing students.[7]

Catholic architecture and images changed in the later twentieth century.
In 1916, for example, the Alexian Brothers' hospital entranceway had several
plaster statues, decorative plants, and a ceiling painted with religious images
that promoted the notion of a sacred space. By 1951, it was much simpler: the
chandelier was gone and there was one statue and a plain ceiling. In 1975,
when the Daughters of Charity's new Seton hospital opened in Austin, they
eliminated many of the statues and pictures so characteristic of the era of
devotional Catholicism and adopted an architectural design that took into
account the latest advances in health care research, with several open court-
yards for patients and visitors. A cascading fountain designed by Texas artist
Anne Cofrin graced the front grounds. The more secular message was that a
beautiful waterfall represented "the continuous flow of life. . . . There are few
things more peaceful or soothing than sitting near flowing water in times of
need or thought," Cofrin stated.[8]

Devotions to the saints also declined in the 1950s and 1960s. As church members grew wealthier and clergy more professionalized, priests began to lift behavioral restrictions and soften once-dogmatic doctrines, contributing to the secularization process.[9] Paula Kane applies this theory to the post–Vatican II Catholic Church: its liberalizing tendencies led Church leaders to deemphasize rewards and punishments associated with devotional practice, leading believers to no longer feel the need to perform them. However, Kane also asserts that many of these tendencies began before Vatican II, as women, in particular, increasingly worked outside the home and expanded their income and independence. They no longer needed the comfort associated with devotions.[10]

Religious teachings also changed during this period, as U.S. Church leaders, influenced by the European call for liturgical reform, began criticizing some of these devotions and images. After Vatican II, the heart of Catholic life was the Mass, and devotions to Mary and the saints were seen as distracting.[11] Along with alterations in taste among Catholics, this shift led not only to the construction of new churches but also to redesigns of hospitals and their chapels. Another possible reason for the change in hospital art was hospitals' dependence on federal money and the increase in regulations attached to it. If a hospital used federal money for construction or received Medicare funding, placing religious objects in the building could violate the doctrine of separation of church and state. Over time, however, many hospitals were able to get exemptions from this regulation.

Religious messages Catholic hospitals offered also changed in response to changes in U.S. culture. In the 1920s the number of Catholics in the United States reached approximately twenty million, and their number continued to grow. With the notable assimilation of Catholics into the larger society after World War II, Catholic hospital leaders, like those in churches and education, by the 1960s were promoting an increasingly American ethos. Catholics were no longer outsiders. As individual Catholics assimilated, they conformed more to the spirit and outlook of the non-Catholic world. Philip Gleason sees this as a time of identity crisis, when the Catholic population differed only marginally from U.S. society at large. Catholic scholars in various disciplines were discarding the belief that their faith dictated an approach different from that of non-Catholics in the same fields. All Catholic institutions were founded upon the assumption that Catholics were somehow different; yet as they assimilated and accepted secular American norms, the social reality that had made that assumption seem necessary eroded. Assimilation at the institutional level brought about a reshaping of hospitals and other Catholic institutions to bring them into line with the middle-class paying patients whose needs they served. As Gleason notes, this transformation began before Vatican II, which only accelerated the "loosening of traditional patterns."[12]

One of the changes that Vatican II instituted was its promulgation of *Perfectae Caritatis* (Perfect Charity), the "Constitution on the Renewal of the Religious Life," which called for revisions to the religious congregations' rules. Sisters and brothers abandoned obsolete practices and outdated customs and simplified their religious clothing; sisters' adoption of modified habits significantly affected the identity of the Catholic hospital. For example, on the same day in 1964, all the Daughters of Charity replaced their white-winged cornettes and gray-blue habits, which they had worn for centuries in Europe and since the 1850s in the United States, with a blue habit and a simpler coif. Eventually sisters had the option of wearing modest secular clothing.[13]

Some Catholic schools and schools of nursing changed their names over the years. The Sisters of Mercy who had established Mercy Hospital in Pittsburgh came from Carlow, Ireland, where they had been associated with Saint Patrick's Carlow College in the 1830s. In 1929 they opened Mount Mercy College and in 1969 changed the name to Carlow College.[14] The ethnic ties and Catholic mission remained, but the new name might attract a more secular public.

Mercy Hospital in Chicago exemplifies some of the changes in hospital artwork. In 1976 it was redesigned with specific spiritual motifs to capture the philosophy and purpose of the Sisters of Mercy. After Vatican II, in response to the call for the Catholic Church to be a new presence to the world, the sisters developed the Committee for EASTER (Evaluation and Study to Effect Revelation) in the context of more effective collaboration with the laity and local communities. One of the committee's projects was to develop a slide show for orientation of new personnel that reflected the interconnection of Mercy's history with the multiple artworks displayed throughout the hospital. These symbolized Mercy's philosophy and purpose, such as the *Sermon on the Mount* by Spanish artist Nassio de Valencia, which was based on the ecumenical idea of brotherhood—that all people were the same in the eyes of God. Taken from a biblical story, it served as the theme for the hospital, where all people, rich or poor, religious or not, could come to be healed. Representing Mercy's response to the community's health needs was a ceramic tile of a Sister of Mercy enfolding the Madonna in her arms, who gives her blessing. In the new chapel, the only totally religious area in the hospital, was an abstract mosaic mural suggesting the mystery of Christ. To the artist de Valencia, it provided the feeling of "an aura of abstraction and mystery" that should "exist in God's house."[15]

At Mercy Hospital in Pittsburgh, Sisters Joanne Marie Andiorio, RSM, and Karen Clarke, RSM, constructed a different kind of religious environment. In 1984 they developed a Ministry of Healing in their new hospital that featured chamber music recitals, choral concerts, and liturgical dramas. To affirm the biblical roots of health care, Sister Elizabeth Ann Madden, RSM, worked with a specially commissioned sculptor on *Christ the Healer*, a thirteen-panel, thirty-five-foot sculpture that was placed in the lobby. In 1987, just outside the new main entrance, the sisters commissioned an architectural firm to construct a porte-cochère featuring a mosaic history of Mercy Hospital and its place in the history of Pittsburgh. The chapel was a centerpiece in the new hospital, where Catholic believers could celebrate the Eucharist, or Holy Communion, as part of the Catholic Mass. No distracting statues cluttered it.[16]

But the new lobby featured not the large figure of Christ that had decorated the main entrance for years but the novel symbol of a pineapple as a sign of hospitality, which was incorporated into a fountain to make the entrance a more tranquil place. While Catholic hospitals before 1950 tapped a rich material culture of art and devotions that Catholic patients would have readily recognized, Mercy's pineapple theme of the 1980s carried a more secular message.

The most important change in Catholic hospitals in the latter part of the twentieth century was the decline in the number of brothers and sisters in all institutions across the United States. No longer were they highly visible in their hospitals twenty-four hours a day, seven days a week. As lay involvement in administration grew, more lay nurses were hired, less on the basis of their commitment to the hospital's religious philosophy than on their educational credentials and skill.[17]

The Alexian Brothers of Chicago

The Alexian Brothers Hospital and School of Nursing in Chicago illustrates these kinds of ongoing changes in religious, ethnic, and gender representations going on around the country. In an era of secularization in midcentury, the brothers linked religion to the gendering of nursing as masculine, devoting themselves to responding to special needs of men. Tensions arose as they updated their ideals of religious service and, sometimes painfully, claimed a new identity based on professional and technological expertise.

The German immigrant community in Chicago was particularly conscious of its origins, which led to a preference for German institutions and the German language and generous support of the Alexian Brothers' hospital. Brother Bonaventure Thelan, CFA, who established the Chicago hospital, came from Germany, as did the other brothers in the early years. When Brother Bonaventure arrived, of the hundred thousand Catholics in Chicago, twenty thousand were German. Located in a German neighborhood, Alexian Brothers Hospital drew mostly patients of German origin, along with men from dozens of other ethnic groups.[18] As the *Chicago Tribune* noted in August 1880, the institution wore the "stamp of decided German character"; patients could eat German food and obtain German Nauheim baths.[19] Admissions demographics changed over time: more U.S.-born patients were admitted, second-generation German Americans moved to the suburbs, and U.S.-born men joined the congregation. As Lawrence Davidson notes: "If the flow of new German immigrants into the city was somehow disrupted, the American identity of the later generations would quickly predominate." These changes affected the "German nature of the hospital, with its primary use of the German language, food, and customs." World War I especially enhanced the Americanization of the brothers; they began integrating the English language into their hospital, but a complete shift to English did not occur until the 1930s.[20]

As the ethnic identity of their group changed over time, the brothers still maintained a distinct Catholic identity in the institutional context of their hospital, where patients experienced the Divine by interacting with religious men. In 1951, the hospital's annual report announced that "while the physical care of patients at Alexian Brothers Hospital is always of great importance, the Hospital is primarily a Religious Institution." The chapel was located on the second floor, but it was readily accessible to patients from the third and fourth floors. The brothers also kept Catholic literature in all the parlors.[21]

While brothers' and sisters' religious clothing was a physical representation of religion, it was mediated by gender and ethnic differences. It appears, for example, that the Alexian Brothers wore black habits for hospital work longer than did most women's nursing communities. At a Catholic Hospital Association (CHA) meeting in 1920, Catholic sister nurses and their male superiors discussed the idea of nuns wearing washable white habits instead of the traditional black ones—physicians preferred the washable clothes to maintain asepsis. While many of the sisters agreed to the change, others resisted, viewing their religious habits as an expression of the differences not only among religious congregations but also between sisters and secular nurses. They felt that to change it would interfere with community traditions and acquiesce to secular demands.[22] But not until sometime after World War II do the brothers appear in white religious garb in their photographs, a change likely the result of the postwar modernization of U.S. hospitals in general, as well as of the growing number of seculars entering the Alexian Brothers' nursing program.[23]

Another way the brothers represented religion to the public was through their nursing practices. They gave prime consideration to the spiritual needs of all patients. In addition to accompanying patients to Mass in the hospital chapel, they emphasized in their 1950 annual report that every one of the six thousand men admitted that year received a visit from the chaplain and a "simple prayer card and was asked to pray every day." Religious devotions in that era were particularly associated with women, but the brothers employed them in their hospital, for example, holding rosary devotions every evening in the chapel.[24]

Catholic clergy, however, constructed an image of nursing that was distinctly feminine. When the Sisters of Providence inaugurated their School of Nursing in Seattle in 1907 for both religious and secular women, Seattle bishop E. J. O'Dea claimed that "nursing was a vocation suited to women on account of their gentle and sympathetic nature" and advised the newly admitted women to "resolve from the very outset to give of their best, after the example of Him 'who went about doing good.'"[25] The clergy wrote advice manuals for women in Catholic schools of nursing that instructed them to be feminine and pious. In the 1930s, Father Alphonse Schwitalla, the president of the CHA, published his view that women nursing students should be submissive, and that their natural nurturing qualities should be cultivated in schools of nursing.[26]

Catholic and non-Catholic nursing schools developed within a cultural framework that saw caring as part of women's role with families and communities.[27] Since the nineteenth century in Europe and the United States, most nursing was done by women, who were regarded as natural-born healers and caretakers. Yet between 1886 and 1929, eight schools of nursing for men opened in the United States: the School of Male Nurses at Blackwell's Welfare Island, New York (1886); McLean Hospital School of Nursing for Men in Waverly, Massachusetts (1886); Mills Training School for Men at Bellevue Hospital in New York City (1888); Saint Vincent Hospital School for Men, also in New York (1888); the Alexian Brothers Hospital School of Nursing in Chicago (1898); Philadelphia's Pennsylvania Hospital School of Nursing (1914);

the Alexian Brothers Hospital School of Nursing in St. Louis (1928); and Saint Joseph's Hospital School of Nursing in New York City (1929).[28] In addition to these programs, until well into the twentieth century, many male nurses graduated from nursing schools connected with psychiatric hospitals.[29] In 1966, a statement by Brother Maurice Wilson, CFA, director of the Alexian Brothers School of Nursing for men, challenged the dominance of the female in most gender analyses of nursing: "There is a place for a masculine character in a predominantly feminine profession."[30] Indeed, men's pursuit of nursing and their representation to the public complicated the idea that nursing was only for women.[31]

Male Caregiving

Care was an essential component of nursing, the Alexian Brothers' chosen ministry. It included tending sick men physically, psychologically, and spiritually. The hospital excelled in departments geared toward men's frequent medical needs, such as urology, neurology, orthopedics, and physical therapy. The brothers' psychiatric facility in St. Louis extended their long ministry of caring for the mentally ill, and in a setting where men nurses had traditionally worked in large numbers. By the 1940s and 1950s, the Alexian Brothers Hospital in Chicago was particularly well known for the care of industrial and genitourinary injuries.[32]

Although the feminist movement provided perspectives of caring that celebrated gender differences, questions persist as to who the caretakers in our culture should be.[33] A particularly influential book by feminist Carol Gilligan appeared in 1982, arguing that caring was something women always did and should continue to do, reinforcing the traditional association of caring with women and buttressing age-old stereotypes. Nel Noddings, a professor of philosophy and education, suggested that caring was a feminine quality but did not have to be gender based. In the midnineties, Julia Wood examined the discursive practices that structured understandings of women and care. She illustrated how Western cultures had strong gender prescriptions, with girls and women expected to be caring and boys and men competitive and assertive. She theorized that "care, like any human activity, is constructed through the discourses of a culture," and that "it is in and through communication that we come to understand our own nature as well as what different interests, activities, and feelings mean and for whom they are 'appropriate.'"[34]

To analyze the notion that caring or other traits are gender specific, one must consider multiple categories that intersect with gender, such as social

class, race, and sexual orientation.[35] Religion is also a consideration. The
Alexian Brothers pursued a religious life with vows of poverty, chastity, and
obedience; a communal lifestyle; and a mission of health care and evangelization. As members of a religious order, they acted upon the traditional religious spirit of self-abnegation, charity, modesty, and humility. Although these
may appear to be the quintessence of feminine traits, all monastic orders of
men and women developed religious identities based on obedience and submission of the will.[36]

Secularization and Professionalization

As the Alexian Brothers maintained a religious identity in their hospitals,
they also embraced modernization. Their hospitals became models of modern technology and architecture. New buildings with clean, shining operating rooms were images that spoke of success and the promise of scientific
achievements, positive images hospitals needed in the increasingly competitive marketplace. In the first part of the twentieth century, as science was
transforming the U.S. hospital, the Alexian Brothers' annual reports for the
Chicago hospital emphasized to physicians and prospective patients that
hospital personnel would practice scientific medicine.[37] It was important to
showcase the compatibility of science and religion, and brothers had photographs taken of them in their religious garb working in areas such as operating rooms and pharmacies to represent themselves as proud members of the
scientific professions of nursing and medicine. Other photographs emphasized activities associated with masculinity: men working in technical areas
such as x-ray departments and physical therapy. These aspiring professionals,
albeit religious, viewed themselves as participants in the expanding world of
hospital medicine. At the same time, the patients admitted to the hospital
received a high standard of care, with the brothers continually updating their
skills through their nursing school.

The Alexian Brothers Hospital School of Nursing incorporated in 1898,
and, as in similar schools, physicians initially provided lectures. In 1899 a
secular nurse, Mr. Hearst, from Mills Training School for Men in New York
was hired as superintendent, although he stayed only a year. The State of Illinois accredited the school in 1925, and the next year witnessed the first class
of brothers to take qualifying exams to become registered nurses. Whereas
their students could obtain psychiatric experience at their St. Louis hospital,
the brothers offered only a general curriculum in Chicago. As nursing standards rose and science and technology expanded in the twentieth century,

the School of Nursing kept pace, requiring more intensive coursework, setting higher admission standards, and giving licensure examinations.[38]

Certain brothers, however, opposed the changes in the school and the growing secularization that came from state regulation. They also objected to the potential corrupting influence of secular students. In the early twentieth century, physicians periodically raised the possibility of enrolling secular students in the school to meet the hospital's need for more nurses, but as one historian noted, seculars did not fit into the closed unit that the brothers had created, in which strict monastic rules insulated the men from seculars.[39] Although in 1927, physicians convinced the brothers to admit four seculars, thereafter the brothers kept the school open only to brothers. Noted in a School of Nursing diary are the minutes of a board of trustees meeting in January 1929, when the brothers decided against admitting any more seculars to the program. "That secular nurses would be a great help in our hospital is undoubtedly true, but to have them train with the novices is a question open to discussion; it has some points not desirable."[40] During these years, tensions escalated between Old and New World ideas. On the one hand, the congregation's leaders in Aachen, Germany, insisted on respect for authority, religious tradition, and loyalty to the congregation, and many of the brothers in Chicago were grounded in this vision. On the other hand, reformers in the U.S. congregation focused on responding to the needs of the situation in that country, which included respect for the values of democracy and education.[41] One of the leaders of the school was concerned that the brothers would consider the nursing program merely "good enough for our young men. This idea would be a big mistake. There is nothing too good for these young men in the educational line for on them the future of the Congregation depends." Indeed, he advocated that the brothers be as professional as their secular counterparts.[42]

While the U.S. brothers remained legally tied to the centralized authority structures in Germany until the 1940s, they continued to Americanize professionally. Brothers earned their baccalaureate degrees and eventually served as officers in professional organizations, both secular and religious.[43] But conflicts between the traditional and the new persisted all along the way. The traditionalists resisted what they viewed as the pernicious trends of New World secularism and modernism, and they disapproved of nonreligious, academic goals. As an example of the sometimes unhappy results of these conflicting views, in 1932 at a General Chapter meeting in Aachen, the brothers decided that novices would do their novitiate in Signal Mountain,

Tennessee, to insulate them from secular influences.[44] When this decision was implemented in 1938, it made the novices unavailable as student nurses in Chicago when the hospital faced a serious nursing shortage. As hospital admissions had decreased during the Great Depression, the small number of nursing brothers and students had kept up with hospital requirements, but the patient load had increased toward the end of the thirties. The brothers would have to choose between religious tradition and daily staffing needs.[45]

The Alexian leaders held an important meeting on January 12, 1939, for the express purpose of "discussing the advisability of accepting secular nurses into the school of nursing." After much discussion the brothers decided to admit them the following September. They also affiliated with DePaul University so students could take biological and physical science courses at DePaul, with the option of applying the credits toward a baccalaureate degree. In the fall of 1939, the brothers admitted thirty-three seculars (although only twenty-seven actually registered). Still emphasizing the importance of religion, they recorded each student's religious affiliation; twenty were Catholic.[46]

The nursing shortage during World War II was potentially devastating to a hospital in which men were the only nurses. The draft loomed large in 1941, and the brothers repeatedly appealed to the draft board for deferments for their students. Fearing a huge loss of students and nurses, the brothers recruited conscientious objectors, a move that brought them into further contact with the secular world. Under the Selective Training and Service Act of 1940, thousands of men were classified 4-E, conscientious objector, and drafted into "work of national importance."[47] Eventually, as part of the Civilian Public Service, the Selective Service offered these pacifist conscriptees to the American Hospital Association. It was from this organization that the brothers requested a unit of workers. Seventy-five men went through their accelerated course in practical nursing and worked in the hospital from 1941 until the end of the war. Sixty-three did actual nursing work, giving baths and backrubs, taking vital signs, making beds, charting patient's conditions, and assisting with admissions and discharges. The others assisted in specialized departments or administration.[48] Eleven became students in the three-year nursing program and graduated. After graduation, half planned to go to medical school, a more traditional profession for men. The others remained in nursing until their retirement.

These men came from Mennonite, Quaker, Church of the Brethren, and Catholic organizations. Describing the religious influence of his nursing education at the Alexian Brothers Hospital, one graduate wrote: "Due to the religious atmosphere and the type of personnel found in the hospital," the conscientious objectors were "more easily accepted here than in some other areas of the population." To him, their work was superior because they had better attitudes and were more willing to do the "extras" for patients. Nursing was a welcome outlet for his pacifism, as opposed to the destruction of war.[49]

While the school stopped admitting students for two years during World War II, it reached its maximum enrollment after the war's conclusion when many servicemen returned. Between September 1945 and February 1947, eighty-eight students enrolled, including some who had served as medics in the military. A few left due to the difficulty of their studies coupled with the school's rigid discipline, but most persevered. By 1950 the nursing school had seventy-two students, eleven brothers and sixty-one seculars, many who were training under the GI Bill of Rights.[50] Afterward, the school's atmosphere changed significantly.

Masculine Representations

The Alexian Brothers Hospital and its School of Nursing were masculine settings where men cared for other men. At the same time, the congregation's members inculcated their philosophy of nursing into their students through monastic rituals for the brothers and spiritual retreats that later were required of all Catholic students, both secular and religious. Secular men's reasons for entering the nursing program varied. Many believed they were called to the nursing profession just as others might be called to the ministry. Several had mothers or sisters who were nurses. One man argued that "a man better understands a man and therefore is better able to help him back to the road to health." The desire to care for others was a recurring theme; most voiced their reasons for going into nursing as a felt "sense of duty to [their] fellow men." One student noted that in nursing, "by easing human suffering, we are fulfilling a command: 'Heal the sick.'"[51]

Christine Williams and Robin Leidner both argue that men's need to interpret their work as manly is greater than women's need to see their work as feminine.[52] Cinzia Solari asserts, however, that "gender dissonance does not mean that there is no room for variation in gendered interpretations of feminized work." Furthermore, workers often interpret their work "in ways that support their gender identities;" for others to recognize this interpretation as valid, however, requires institutional support.[53] The Alexian Brothers Hospital and School of Nursing provided this support. It allowed students to renegotiate notions of masculinity to include nursing as manly work that followed a Christian calling.

In the 1940s, as the nursing shortage forced the Alexian Brothers to attract more seculars to their school, their public marketing began focusing on masculine aspects of nursing. Just as they built religion into their physical surroundings, they masculinized the spaces of the nursing school, adding pool tables, a large swimming pool, and a boxing ring for student tournaments.[54] Other sports teams such as volleyball and football formed (see figure 8). The image of the male nurse portrayed by these activities showed that nursing was not strictly a feminine profession.

The 1942 valedictory address illustrates how men nurses used gender distinctions to gain acceptance for their work. The speaker argued that men should be accepted as nurses in the Army and Navy Nurse Corps. At that time, men who were registered nurses could enlist or be drafted, but they could not be assigned as nurses. The war provided an opportunity for men nurses to press their claims to professional equality with women in the military.

Noting the uncertainty of the future, the valedictorian asked: "In view of the need for competent nurses by the government, must I disregard all that I

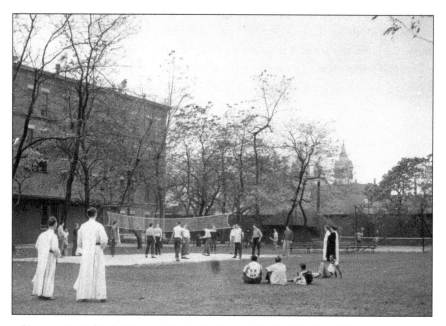

Figure 8   Volleyball team, Alexian Brothers School of Nursing, Chicago, ca. 1951.
Courtesy Alexian Brothers Provincial Archives, Arlington Heights, Illinois.

have learned in training, in order to take up a gun? As a registered man nurse, would I be of no value as such to my country?" Revealing the insecurities some men nurses had over the perceived status of female nurses compared to their own, the speaker distinguished himself and his fellow students as being not only different from but also better than women in some areas, although he did not elaborate: "Whether or not the 'ladies of the cloth' will admit it, the fact still remains that the man nurse is more competent than they in many situations which arise in medical services—that he can step in where the angels fear to tread. . . . Certain aspects of contemporary hospital service have only too obviously proven it." He closed his address with a reference to religion: "Nursing, when properly motivated, is one of the finest ways to show that Christ-like love for our fellow men."[55] Gender stereotypes trumped need, however. Federal law and a preference for female nurses prevented men from receiving reserve commissions in the Army Nurse Corps until 1955, and they did not obtain full military commissions until 1966 during the Vietnam War. In 1964, men entered the Navy Nurse Corp.[56]

Sexuality issues were one of the potentially negative influences that secular students could bring to the school. Although archival sources are silent about heterosexual and homosexual matters, this was a time when the public perceived gender roles as distinctly separate. To counter any public suspicion that men who chose nursing were either homosexual or effeminate, the Alexian Brothers went to great lengths to convey the image of the male nurse as a virile professional. A section in the school yearbook entitled "Memorable Events" described energetic men engaging in all manner of activities such as coeducational dances and parties, class picnics, and initiation rites. One graduate recalled in September 3, 1952: "Faces smeared with shoe polish, lipstick and a generous supply of tape . . . clothes on backwards . . . greased volley ball . . . mass calisthenics."[57] The message was clear: in this all-male school, active men participated in sports and other masculine and heterosexual activities. This countered any stereotype of nursing schools as necessarily feminine spaces.

The valedictory address in 1955 suggests how language and communication were shaped by gender and religion among these students. In celebrating the role of men in nursing, the graduate elaborated on the characteristics of a "good nurse": generosity of spirit, patience, cheerfulness, self-sacrifice, and effacement—qualities some consider feminine. But he also listed the traditionally masculine characteristics of executive ability, courage, and willingness to submit to strict discipline and hard work.[58] Clearly, through their training school experiences with the Alexian Brothers, these men developed a special religious and professional identity as nurses. As they underscored their skills, they also framed their work as a way of serving God. They embraced qualities usually portrayed as feminine, but they gave the clear message that men as well as women could personify them. However, in their attempt to broaden social ideas about masculinity, they identified other qualities in themselves more commonly associated with men, such as bravery, executive skills, and discipline.

When the Alexian Brothers built a new nursing school building in 1955, they admitted larger classes and increased their faculties, and the school obtained full National League for Nursing accreditation. In 1962, thirteen full-time faculty members and eight lecturers educated a graduating class of forty-two, the largest in the school's history and one of the largest classes in any men's nursing school in the country.[59] Many students were likely attracted by the school's publications that stressed that men nurses were more apt to advance to specialized fields such as anesthesia, education, and supervisory work.

By the mid 1960s, men were entering the Alexian nursing program with specific career paths in mind. Williams argues that today, nursing instructors often shunt men nurses onto administrative paths and into highly technical roles; students' experiences in the Alexian Brothers school serves as a historical parallel.[60] Several men planned to use nursing as a stepping-stone to becoming physicians, a traditionally masculine ambition for acquiring education and power. Gender was a structuring force for other positions the secular graduates assumed. A 1966 survey showed that most were working in prestigious and high-paying positions: 42 percent in anesthesia and 24 percent in administration. Others were doing typical "men's work," with 22 percent serving in the military and 12 percent working in industrial and psychiatric nursing. Floor nursing, which required more intimate hands-on work, attracted only 18 percent. There the men worked as head nurses and staff nurses. Only 6 percent were clinical instructors.[61]

After five years of discussions with experts in the field, in 1969 the Alexian Brothers decided to close the school. Although, through affiliations with other hospitals, they were offering students specialized maternity and pediatrics courses, the last yearbook noted that "four-year university and college programs are better equipped to produce the highly-specialized nurse that is needed today, and this is especially true of the man in nursing."[62] This last phrase is telling. In the eyes of the Alexian instructors, higher-education credentials separated men nurses from women, allowing the men to maintain their masculine identities as they worked in a female-dominated job. Thus, as the Alexian Brothers and their students attempted to undo gender stereotypes in a variety of publications, they maintained gender differences by adhering to the idea that men nurses held certain advantages over women nurses.

At the school's closing, Brother Maurice noted that the goal of the school had not been "to make the nursing profession masculine." Rather, throughout its seventy-one years of existence, it had aimed to gain society's acceptance of men in nursing: "When society questioned the reason why a man went into nursing, when the armed forces refused to recognize this man, and even when the professional organization was quiet in its acceptance of men into its ranks, the Alexian Brothers were quietly but persistently promoting and encouraging men to move into the hospital field." To this end, the brothers provided opportunities for 779 men to graduate in nursing. Of this number, 621 were seculars. In the final yearbook, the men represented their masculine identities to the public in photos of graduates serving in the military, working in highly technical areas of acute care and anesthesia, becoming physicians, and posing with their families.[63]

The story of the Alexian Brothers and the men they educated is a testament to the power of religion and gender in medical and nursing history. These men confronted the often-held notion that religious pursuits and masculinity were incongruent. They carved out a system that recognized caring as a responsibility not only of women but also of men. As they asserted that their paid work was a Christian calling, they renegotiated prevailing ideas about masculinity.[64] Although the secular students felt called to their profession, they also embraced it as a career and therefore had no misgivings about being paid for the service they rendered. In this manner, they blended the religious calling with secular values.

In so doing, men nurses navigated an array of representations, from nurse, to school administrator, to soldier, to religious person, to professional practitioner of scientific medicine. It was the Alexian Brothers' religious institutions that set the conditions for the way religious and gender identities were woven together. In some ways, the fears of the traditionalists came true after seculars entered the nursing program. As seculars outnumbered religious in the school, publications displayed images that had as much to do with masculine as religious roles. These self-representations in the masculine spaces of the hospital and nursing school were designed to debunk stereotypes of feminine men, and they challenged traditional gender boundaries in nursing.

Conclusion

The broad cultural issues of religion and gender in health care are complex. The Alexian Brothers reenvisioned the notion of masculinity as they pushed against the gendered boundaries of nursing. As they negotiated their gender identities, the Alexian Brothers defined nursing as Christian work. This influenced the secular men who entered the hospital and nursing school. At the same time, seculars represented themselves to the public in ways that often separated them from female nurses. By the mid-twentieth century, men graduates typically followed the traditionally masculine paths of nursing administration, anesthesia, highly technical roles, and military nursing.[65]

Public representations were increasingly important not only in Catholic schools of nursing but also in the twentieth-century hospital. Stevens has noted that "hospitals . . . are affirming and defining mirrors of the culture in which we live. . . . Through the scope and style of the buildings, the organizational 'personality' of the institution, and the underlying meaning of the whole enterprise," hospitals "beam back to us" values that owners want to display.[66] Catholic architecture and images changed over the later twentieth century as indicators of changes not only in religious beliefs, but also in ideas about what a hospital should be, who should run it, and whom it should serve. Before the 1960s sisters and brothers used religious objects in their hospitals and schools of nursing to tell the world around them that they were Catholic. With increasing secularization, changes in theology, and modifications in individual taste, Catholics hospital leaders displayed more ecumenical symbols to assist them in marketing to non-Catholics and a growing middle class. With Catholic symbols blending with ecumenical images, non-Catholics would not feel uncomfortably surrounded by religious icons.

Patients entering a Catholic hospital today can still find familiar religious symbols that depict the faith, but the hospital environment is acceptably appealing to both Catholics and non-Catholics. It serves as a valuable connection to the worlds of special economic interests and of belief systems. All these entities interacted to reconfigure the U.S. Catholic hospital of the late twentieth century.

Chapter 4

Regardless of Color, Race, Creed, or Financial Status

In 1955, Brother Constantine Krohn, administrator of Alexian Brothers Hospital in Chicago, explained to twenty-two Catholic hospital representatives from the Archdiocese of Chicago the Alexian Brothers' decision to desegregate their hospital and the positive benefits it had brought. Integration, he noted, enabled the Alexian Brothers to fulfill more completely the objectives for which their hospital was established—"to care for the sick regardless of color, race, creed, or financial status." This decision, said Krohn, led to better patient care, since the patients were placed in nursing units on the basis only of their diagnosis.[1] From their inception in the United States, Catholic hospitals had claimed to care for all those in need, regardless of race, creed, or ability to pay.[2] However, in parts of the country, Catholic institutions either did not admit minority patients or segregated them in private rooms or older wings; black physicians could not practice at all. Because the passage of Medicare and Medicaid in 1965 prohibited discrimination in hospitals and other public places that received federal funding, the discussion here focuses on the years before 1970.[3]

Religion, race, gender, economics, and region worked together to shape the history of hospitals. During the first half of the twentieth century, Jim Crow laws in the southern and border states legally sanctioned racial segregation, especially of blacks, in all public facilities. In Washington State, where it was illegal to discriminate on the basis of race, the antidiscrimination law was almost never enforced; while not as severely as in the South, Seattle practiced segregation in housing and other areas, not only for blacks but also for Asians.[4] John McGreevy and Thomas Sugrue both detail the abundance of racial tensions in northern cities, where large numbers of blacks had migrated in the 1940s, arguing that some neighborhoods for blacks and whites were significantly more segregated than those in the South.[5] By 1970, racial segregation characterized U.S. urban areas, as blacks concentrated in inner cities surrounded by predominantly white suburbs.[6]

In the early and mid-twentieth century, as white hospitals and schools of nursing denied access to black patients, physicians, and nurses, the black community created separate health care institutions.[7] In 1944, 124 hospitals catered exclusively to black patients in the United States, and 20 had schools of nursing. While efforts toward racial integration after World War II targeted education, voting rights, and desegregation of public places such as restaurants, a less publicized issue was discrimination in hospitals.[8]

When the Hill-Burton Act passed into law in 1946, it provided federal funds for the construction of hospitals, nursing homes, mental health facilities, and public health centers all across the country; half the new institutions were built in the South. The program maintained a "separate but equal" clause, asserting that blacks should have services of equal quality to whites,' either in all-black hospitals or in segregated wards in white institutions. These federally sponsored facilities increased the care available to many black and indigent patients, but the Hill-Burton Act failed to end racial discrimination in hospitals. Not for two more decades was full compliance with integration made a condition of federal aid in all health care facilities, as a result of the Supreme Court's ruling in *Simkins v. Cone* in 1963, the Civil Rights Act of 1964, and Medicare and Medicaid laws in 1965.[9]

A 1957 study of national trends in hospital integration found that only 25 percent of both northern and southern hospitals had black physicians on their staffs. All the sample hospitals in the South were still segregated, as were 13 percent of hospitals in the North. Furthermore, in both regions, restrictive practices rather than full integration were common, including observing a quota of black admissions, making only single private rooms available to blacks, and admitting blacks only to semi-private rooms occupied by another black patient. Some hospitals, especially in large metropolitan areas, segregated blacks in overcrowded wards, basements, or attics.[10]

In 1940, the annual mortality rate for whites was 10.8 per 1,000 population and 13.8 for nonwhites ("white" and "nonwhite" are terms the Census Bureau was using in 1960, when these figures were published). While it had decreased in 1960 for all populations, a discrepancy still existed, at 9.5 for whites and 10.1 for nonwhites. Blacks also lagged behind whites in longevity and infant mortality: the life expectancy of whites was 70.6 years, of nonwhites, 63.6 years. In 1960 the national infant mortality rate was 22.9 per 1,000 live births for white babies under one year of age and 43.2 for nonwhite babies. Regional discrepancies also existed. In Alabama, where fewer health care services were available to everyone, the infant mortality rate for whites was 24.9 compared to 45 for nonwhites; in Washington, it was 22.7 for whites and 36.7 for nonwhites.[11]

Catholic hospitals integrated over time. The Franciscan Sisters of the Immaculate Conception from Little Falls, Minnesota, under the auspices of the Capuchin fathers, began operating Saint Anthony's Hospital in Milwaukee as a fully integrated, nonsegregated facility in 1931. In 1951, Sister Helen Bauerback, a Sister of St. Joseph in Wheeling and head of Saint Francis Hospital, hired three black nurses, prompting twenty white nurses to quit. Sister Helen stood firm on her decision, and sisters from other West Virginia hospitals came to staff the hospital. That same year the Daughters of Charity's all-white Saint Vincent Maternity Hospital in Kansas City opened its doors to patients of all races. By 1953, the hospital staff was biracial, with thirty-nine black doctors and a ratio of 3:1 black to white patients. In Cairo, Illinois, in the 1950s and 1960s, the Sisters of the Holy Cross battled doctors and city leaders when the nuns admitted blacks and hired black workers. In 1954, they had 6 black physicians of 189 at their hospital in South Bend, Indiana; they also hired Asian physicians.[12] Other Catholic hospitals were slow to integrate, and it was not until the late 1960s, either by law or by request from religious authorities, that they eliminated segregation altogether.

Chicago: "Submit in Humility to Segregation and Discrimination"

The experience of hospitals in Chicago exemplifies the protracted struggle against segregated health care institutions. In that city, medical and nursing needs for blacks mushroomed after the great migrations before and after World War I. In 1900, the black population in Chicago was 30,000; by the mid 1930s, it had grown to more than 235,000. Between 1940 and 1950, it increased from 277,731 to 492,265, a growth of 77 percent, as blacks took advantage of new manufacturing jobs in the city.[13] As early as the 1920s, the *Chicago Defender*, the country's largest black newspaper, was protesting the exclusion of black patients and doctors from white hospitals. Vanessa Northington Gamble describes discrimination against blacks by the University of Chicago clinics in the 1930s and 1940s.[14] At that time, only Cook County General Hospital, Michael Reese, and Provident Hospital, the first black-controlled health care institution in the country, admitted blacks, even though there were twenty-five Catholic hospitals in the city. Many of the Catholic institutions operated in changing neighborhoods that had seen white Catholic European immigrants flee to the suburbs and blacks move in. Catholic clergy and laypersons sometimes led movements to keep blacks out of white neighborhoods.[15]

Several voices protested against hospital segregation, including that of Maude Johnston, a prominent black Catholic who in 1944, after a serious myocardial infarction, wrote to Samuel Cardinal Stritch, Chicago's archbishop, regarding her experience at the Catholic Mercy Hospital: "Dr. Hellsmith, over the phone, advised my husband to bring me, at once, to the hospital. When I arrived there, he said he was sorry, and that he thought I was somebody else. And then followed a conversation in which I said that I was willing and able to pay for my room. But he maintained that the Mercy Hospital just did not take colored people." She reiterated that the sister in the admissions office said that the board was going to discuss the question of accepting blacks to the hospital, but a decision had not yet been made. "In the meantime, my husband and two relatives put me back in the car. And upon arriving at Cook County Hospital I was given Extreme Unction, not being expected to live."[16] The topic of admitting blacks came up again at the 1949 meeting of Mercy's board of trustees, which consisted of seven sisters. They were "not yet ready to take in" blacks at that time, although they had long cared for blacks in the Mercy Dispensary.[17] Cardinal Stritch successfully convinced the Sisters of Mercy to lift their racial ban in the hospital.[18]

As in other parts of the country, hospital opportunities for black physicians, interns, and residents were limited in Chicago. In 1950 Dr. A. M. Mercer, president of the Cook County Physicians Association for black doctors, asserted that black Catholics could not enter a Catholic hospital like other Catholics, particularly targeting Chicago's Catholic hospitals: "They *can enter* provided they submit in humility to segregation and discrimination. . . . A white Atheist doctor has a much better chance of joining their staffs than a qualified Catholic Negro doctor" [emphasis in original].[19] Indeed, in the late 1950s, Mercy Hospital accepted medical residents from Turkey, Iran, the Philippines, Cuba, Peru, Brazil, and Lithuania, but no blacks. By then, the hospital was admitting some blacks as patients; the *1952 Annual Report* listed 400, or 4 percent of total admissions. Of all admissions, 191 were Jewish, 7,457 Catholic, and 2,373 Protestant.[20]

Censure of racial discrimination mounted in the late 1950s. Voices raised against it included the Catholic Interracial Council of Chicago (CIC) and a group at Friendship House, an organization established to promote interracial justice. Both were active in conducting educational activities to change the thinking of nuns, priests, and the laity on issues of race. Cardinal Stritch also took an aggressive stance against hospital discrimination, writing labor and civil rights activist Monsignor Daniel Cantwell in October 1955: "When I came to Chicago I was a bit shocked at the attitude of some of our hospitals." At a conference of hospital administrators sponsored by the CIC, Stritch delivered a strong speech on racism. "Charity embraces all and where these ugly distinctions obtain they have been justified on the grounds that the privately controlled hospital, has to have patients in order to enable it to do its charity, and it cannot so extend its charity that it will become impossible to do any charity," he said. "[This] argument is getting less and less force. And courageous action will make that argument entirely ineffective and without weight."[21]

Stritch supported a study on race issues sponsored by the CIC and Friendship House, and the picture was not bright. One sister administrator responded that her hospital did not typically admit blacks. Occasionally they got transfers from Cook County if it was overcrowded, but they segregated them because they anticipated complaints from whites. The study found only one hospital, the Alexian Brothers, that admitted patients regardless of race. A sister from another hospital commented that they had no trouble because they kept blacks in private rooms, even if it meant the patients had to pay private room rates. Most hospitals hired blacks, but only as nurses' aides, kitchen help, or laundrywomen. All excluded black physicians, while only a few reported black registered nurses on staff.[22] In 1956, a city ordinance passed that forbade racial exclusion in all hospitals; to ensure compliance, a group from the CIC visited each Catholic facility in the archdiocese. A follow-up report noted that Catholic hospitals faced a moral dilemma, as too many of them did not serve their local communities. It indicted sister superiors for their lack of courage in fighting contemporary racial norms; the nuns "know that sick people in need in the local community are not being served because of race. They have no [black] staff doctors nor do many of their doctors take Negro patients." The segregation of black patients in separate rooms was the result of submission to pressure from white doctors who did not want blacks in the same room as their white patients, the report claimed. "The nuns have lost control of their hospitals to the staff doctors. By canon law a Catholic hospital must be owned and controlled by the Catholic order. However, in actual practice, control on the policy level is directed by the staff. Many staff doctors have the sisters convinced that they would quit or lose all their patients if the hospital had Negro doctors. We know that they wouldn't lose patients and doctors need staff positions to make money. They won't quit."[23]

Other barriers to Catholic hospital desegregation were economic. Some Catholic hospitals were reluctant to accept blacks because of a general suspicion that they could not pay their bills.[24] These institutions relied on white doctors to bring in patients, and many of the physicians were not willing to treat blacks. Because of their financial dependence on the doctors, the sisters were afraid to challenge them. They had learned what Amy Koehlinger has called "strategic silence and strategic complicity."[25]

Members of the CIC voiced the belief that the Chicago hospital situation would change in the near future, when religious congregations might indeed comply because of their concern to give service to all. In addition, as more industries provided medical insurance plans for employees, the CIC thought that industrial leaders and unions would pressure hospital boards and physicians to care for all their workers. Industrial leaders would probably not contribute endowment funds to hospitals that would not care for their black employees who had hospital and health insurance.[26]

When the CIC went to Saint Bernard's Hospital, it found that the sister administrator had posted copies of the new city ordinance on the medical staff bulletin board and in the emergency room. Copies were also to be given to the physicians and admission personnel. Until recently, blacks had been assigned to private rooms. The hospital did have black registered nurses and technicians. While the children's ward was integrated, white adults were still being asked whether they were willing to share a semi-private room with a black person. Many whites still objected to integrated rooms, including physicians. The sister administrator claimed she had tried to hire two black doctors, but the white doctors would not have a black doctor on staff. Nor did white doctors admit black patients; rather, blacks usually came to the emergency room, where the sisters admitted them and then assigned them to a physician. In fact, as the local community had changed, most of the white doctors had left the hospital and moved to the suburbs. The sisters had decided to stay because it was a mission area for them. As the sister administrator said: "No need to go overseas when there is a need right here."[27]

Another CIC visit revealed that a specialty hospital for obstetrics and gynecology run by Catholic sisters had Chinese and Japanese physicians on staff but no black doctors or nurses. The sister administrator said that black doctors or nurses would be hired based on their qualifications, not their skin color, but that none had applied. While black patients had been segregated in the past, they were not at the current time. The number of blacks coming to the hospital was increasing and most had insurance and could pay.[28] Another study reported that the three diocesan hospitals in the city had more black physicians than ten other Catholic hospitals put together.[29]

The Alexian Brothers hospital offers some contrast. While the brothers had agreed to admit black candidates into their novitiate in 1920, they reversed their decision six years later.[30] Unlike the administrators of some hospitals, however, the Alexian Brothers eliminated segregation in their facility in 1953 by abolishing their two all-black wards and agreeing to assign patient rooms based solely on diagnosis. Significantly, Brother Constantine noted that there had been a few complaints by the white patients, but the brothers settled the grievances by diplomatically stating their policy and stressing the Christian attitude against segregation.

In the 1950s Catholic schools of nursing, like others in the country, began opening their doors to minorities, although usually only wide enough for one or two to enter. In 1950, one Japanese student and one man were among the seventeen graduates of Seattle University School of Nursing, Providence Unit. The 1954 first-year class for Chicago's Sisters of Mercy's diploma program had one black nurse. And the first black male nursing student graduate in the country, Marcus Walker, completed the Alexian Brothers School of Nursing program in 1952.[31]

Although Brother Constantine played down complaints from patients, the brothers in fact had received criticism from white physicians who objected to the integration policy, fearing a negative reaction from their patients.[32] The doctors tried to get the hospital administration, still composed of brothers at this time, to reverse the decision and almost succeeded. As one historian reports: "One morning before Mass, Father Clement walked to the front of the chapel and delivered a passionate plea that the brothers stick to their guns and not abandon this basically just plan. Whether or nor his words were responsible, the plan went through and worked."[33]

The brothers also followed a nondiscrimination policy in hiring physicians. In 1956 there were two black physicians on staff at Alexian Brothers Hospital. Approximately 10 percent of the patients were black, and the brothers reported that more blacks than whites paid for their care. They also noted that they were "supporting the local conservation board in its efforts to fight a blighted neighborhood. We will remain here if the population changes in its racial character, continuing to serve those we were founded to serve—sick people in our community."[34]

Throughout the 1950s, Chicago's black press continued to report on segregation in public accommodations, including hospitals.[35] In 1958, the *Daily Defender* reported that Chicago still lagged far behind many other cities in eliminating discrimination in hospital admissions and in the percentage of black physicians affiliated with white hospitals. That year, the U.S. Conference of Catholic Bishops finally spoke out against racism in its statement "Discrimination and the Christian Conscience," labeling it a "moral evil" that denied humans their dignity as children of God.[36] The following year only five Catholic hospitals—Alexian Brothers, Mercy, Lewis, Loretto, and Saint Bernard—appointed black physicians to their staffs.[37] In 1961, however, Mercy was one of several Chicago hospitals named in a lawsuit that charged discrimination against black doctors for staff positions. Afterward, the sisters admitted three black physicians to courtesy staff appointments.[38]

Blatant discrimination in Chicago's Catholic hospitals had ended by the late 1960s and 1970s. But questions were being asked about how the government should deal with not-for-profit hospitals that moved to affluent, primarily white suburbs from unprofitable inner-city locations where they had provided care to the poor.[39] As more Catholics entered the middle classes in midcentury and moved from urban ethnic neighborhoods into less ethnic but racially segregated suburbs, they took their schools, churches, and hospitals with them.[40] Many priests encouraged this exodus. In 1956, for example, one priest noted that as many as two and a half million Catholics had transplanted since the 1940s, with predictions that five to eight million more would move to the suburbs in the next two decades. This was an opportunity for the lay apostolate to grow and showcase basic Catholic values of family life in a rapidly secularizing society. The shift was risky, however, as the Catholic Church would not necessarily be the church for the poor anymore. In 1958, sociologist and priest Andrew Greeley noted that while conversion efforts should not neglect the poor, "we must also face the deep and tangled problems that many Catholics are encountering as they become suburbanites."[41] In 1970, a speaker at the Catholic Hospital Association Convention described the problems associated with changing inner-city demographics and called on Catholic hospitals to act as "trailblazers in effecting necessary change" for better medical care for inner-city residents.[42]

Although the Alexian Brothers had originally planned to keep their hospital in the inner-city area where the highest rate of poverty was centered, in 1966 they moved to Elk Grove in the northwestern suburbs. As wealthier whites and blacks had moved out of the city to the suburbs, they had left a core of impoverished blacks, and, as noted earlier, Chicago's inner city had become one of the nation's most segregated areas.[43] The Alexian Brothers hospital's German identity had faded as German American Catholics had assimilated into society at large, and an extensive study by the Chicago Hospital District had shown that the inner-city patients would be absorbed by other hospitals in the area. The brothers did note that the nonwhite patients might have problems with admissions to other hospitals because Alexian Brothers Hospital had taken in such a large number.[44]

While 62.2 percent of whites in Chicago had moved to the suburbs by 1970, only 10 percent of blacks had done so. And as the white population had shifted westward, so had the physicians. A 1973 study noted that poor neighborhoods in the inner city, left with fewer physicians and nurses, had significantly poorer health outcomes.[45]

Viewed strictly from a business perspective, the brothers' choice to relocate their hospital to the suburbs was an understandable, even wise, decision. Yet when one considers their religious calling to minister to those in greatest need, their decision to depart from the inner city likely was a difficult choice for them to make in that it posed a conflict between spiritual ideals and their business pragmatism. In the end, they chose a gray middle ground—to continue their policies of admitting and treating impoverished patients, but in a location populated mainly by affluent citizens.

In professional circles, the status of Alexian Brothers Medical Center increased significantly after its relocation. In 1998, it ranked eleventh in a survey, albeit a controversial one, of eighty-two Chicago hospitals by HCIA, a Baltimore-based health information company. HCIA analyzed data from the federal government that included Medicare cost reports, financial profiles, and market power—the ability to draw patients from outside the hospital service region—in the areas of oncology, cardiology, and orthopedics. It also included morbidity and mortality rates. Saint Bernard Hospital, which had remained in Chicago's South Side Englewood neighborhood, a primarily low-income area, particularly suffered in terms of resources and was rated last. Its leaders noted that the survey did not accurately reflect the hospital's quality of care, because it provided more care with less reimbursement and more obstacles than any other hospital in the city. Noticeably absent from the survey were the hospitals' service missions and admission practices, and patients themselves did not participate.[46] One might speculate that had these components been included, the outcome might well have been different, particularly if the survey respondents represented all socioeconomic levels.

The Sisters of Mercy also kept their hospital in the Near South Side. Differences with the Stritch School of Medicine had affected their decision not to move to Skokie with the medical school in the 1950s, as noted earlier. In addition, neighborhood leaders appealed to the sisters to keep Mercy at its present site to help stabilize the area. Since 1921, they had operated their large dispensary with the Stritch School of Medicine, which provided more than sixty thousand patient visits annually. The dispensary served patients who had limited access to medical services, including a large black population from the surrounding neighborhood. Mercy provided free beds, medicine, x-rays, and other services and facilities.[47] In 1961 the Sisters of Mercy recommitted themselves to their heritage of service to the poor. Their admission policy clarified that "in every case, the care which is given is determined by need of the patient, without regard to sex, race, or color and no particular religious faith is required."[48] As noted earlier, however, the sisters' decision to stay hurt them financially, and they continued to struggle into the twenty-first century.

Pacific Northwest: "Very Happy to Have Him Returned"

Seattle was segregated for much of its early history, excluding people of color from many jobs, neighborhoods, stores, restaurants, and hotels, and from some hospitals. As in other western states, racial discrimination targeted not just blacks but also American Indians, Asians, Mexican Americans, and Jews.[49] As early as 1902, however, the Sisters of Providence admitted blacks into their hospital in Vancouver, Washington, and their records show they continued to do so through the early twentieth century. The majority of patients were Irish, German, Canadian, Swedish, and American-born whites; the sisters had a separate ward for Japanese patients at Providence Saint Vincent's Hospital in Portland, Oregon.[50] At Providence Hospital, Seattle, in 1927, the sisters advertised that "no line is drawn as to race or creed."[51]

An incident of alleged racial discrimination occurred at Seattle's Providence Hospital School of Nursing in 1928 when it denied an American-born Japanese woman admission. At that time, the School of Nursing publications noted that the sisters used "extreme care" in choosing applicants.[52] Whether the denial was based on ethnicity or lack of qualifications is unknown, but it caused widespread outrage in the Japanese American community.[53] The hospital fared better on this score. In 1930, the sisters received letters of thanks for their hospital services from two Jewish rabbis, an archbishop of the Russian Orthodox Church, a black woman who named her baby after Saint Vincent, and a Japanese seaman.[54]

Although the Pacific Northwest was host to a significant and prosperous Japanese community, the Immigration Act in 1924 effectively stopped Japanese immigration to the United States, and the *Seattle Star* began mobilizing public opinion against Japanese and Japanese Americans already in the city. During World War II, more than seven thousand Seattle-area Japanese were sent to resettlement camps, and at war's end the *Seattle Star* published editorials against their return.[55] By contrast, in 1942 the Seattle Council of Churches opposed Japanese evacuation and relocation. In March and May of that year, the Sisters of Providence recorded distressing notes about the evacuations. Catholic priests and clergy of other religious denominations followed their Japanese parishioners to the registration centers and often opened churches in the camps.[56]

Aided by religious organizations and the American Friends Service Committee, the National Japanese American Student Relocation Council organized in 1942 to help relocate students to colleges outside the military zones on the West Coast. The U.S. government also formed a group, the War Relocation Authority, to help interned Japanese and Japanese Americans to become reestablished. With the assistance of these groups, approximately thirty schools of nursing in the United States admitted students of Japanese ancestry in 1944. During World War II, according to the *American Journal of Nursing*, 315 Japanese American women enrolled in nursing programs. Approximately 195 enlisted in the federally funded U.S. Cadet Nursing Corps, and Japanese American men served in the military in the European theater.[57]

When the government rescinded the internment orders in 1945, more protests occurred in Seattle. The Sisters of Providence had employed a Japanese worker at Saint Mary Hospital in Astoria, Oregon, since the 1920s, and he was one of the first Japanese nationals to be released from a federal internment camp in 1945. The sisters immediately reinstated him at his former position of cook, leading some local citizens to boycott Saint Mary's. The sisters, however, wrote that they were "very happy to have him returned." Indeed, his kitchen work relieved the sister in charge of "much labor."[58]

The Japanese constituted the largest minority in Seattle until World War II, when thousands of black workers came to the city for war jobs. Seattle remained prosperous after the war as Boeing Airlines, the city's largest industry, continued to receive lucrative military contracts and commercial

airline orders. Although discrimination in employment and housing persisted, by 1950 blacks in Seattle could get higher wages in several industrial jobs than they could in other parts of the country. Thus, the *Chicago
Defender* urged blacks to leave the Midwest and head for Seattle. The black
population grew by 164 percent during the war and by 169 percent between
1945 and 1960.[59] This influx placed a huge burden on the city's resources,
including its hospitals.

Seattle's NAACP, founded in 1913, was quite active in protesting and fil-
ing lawsuits against racial discrimination in the Northwest. The NAACP's
leadership was particularly prominent on the Seattle Civic Unity Committee.[60] In March 1945, the Christian Friends for Racial Equality in Seattle
called the attention of the Civic Unity Committee to the difficulty blacks
had in obtaining hospital care. Acting on information received through the
State Department of Health, they claimed that the larger hospitals in Seattle,
including Harborview, Columbus, and Providence, received blacks only if
they had private rooms available. The other large hospital, Swedish, did not
admit blacks at all.[61] No records could be found to validate these claims. In
1955, records show that Providence Hospital admitted 16,261 white patients,
429 black patients, and 476 "other."[62]

These accounts make it clear that the sisters' treatment of minorities was
more value driven and inclusive than U.S. societal norms of that era would
dictate. Still, they made pragmatic business decisions that clearly bowed to
public opinion, placing minority patients in segregated hospital wards and
possibly refusing members of minorities admission to nursing schools. There
was no absolute adherence to their religious tenets regarding human equality.
Like some other sisters and brothers running Catholic hospitals, they settled
for the gray area of partial appeasement.

Also like other sisters and brothers, the Sisters of Providence were profoundly influenced by Vatican II. The final document to be promulgated, *Gaudium et Spes* (Joy and Hope), or the "Pastoral Constitution on the Church in
the Modern World," placed the Catholic Church firmly in, rather than apart
from, the world. Article 2 stated: "Therefore, the Council focuses its attention
on the world of men, the whole human family along with the sum of those
realities in the midst of which that family lives."[63] Catholic sisters and brothers came to reject discrimination against men or women or harassment of
them because of their race, color, condition of life, or religion. After Vatican
II the Sisters of Providence in Seattle participated in Masses for civil rights;
and in 1967, ninety-three nuns from their congregation attended a Carl Rogers

Sensitivity Workshop hosted by their hospital. In 1969 the sisters celebrated the Chinese New Year at Providence Hospital, which included showing films about Chinese culture.[64]

Providence Hospital was located near Seattle's Central District, a predominantly black area where, increasingly over the 1960s, blacks felt besieged by deep-seated racism. Despite the growth of Boeing, blacks still experienced job discrimination, which added to the poverty in the Central District. In 1967, for example, the unemployment rate for blacks in Seattle was 10 percent.[65] Because of random violence and attacks on property near the hospital, police came to guard the facility's entrances in 1970. As the sisters' chronicler wrote: "Our black brothers seriously question the sincerity and love of the white man. Because of this, it becomes necessary to protect the innocent."[66]

The persistent poverty continued to generate tensions between blacks and whites. In 1971, the sisters undertook a study of discrimination in their eleven West Coast hospitals. They sent questionnaires to all employees and physicians, asking, "Do you have personal knowledge of any incident of racial discrimination in the hospital?" Only 203, or 3 percent, of the 6,000 responses reported in the affirmative, although employees may not have been truthful, since the owners and administrators of the hospitals were conducting the study. A typical comment was that there were no black registered nurses, with the majority of blacks employed in more menial jobs or those requiring heavy lifting. Others reported less pay for minorities, the separation of white patients on one side of the hall and minorities on the other, the segregation of "hippies," and the separation of black from white babies. Some white patients had insulted minority employees, opposed sharing a room with a minority patient, and objected to care by a minority employee. Whereas some patients complained that white employees did not want to care for black patients, other white employees reported that black patients did not want white nurses. The sixteen white physicians who noted incidents of discrimination cited events such as a retired sister trying to convert a patient to Catholicism and a fellow doctor who was discriminatory. Although the reports were few in number, the sisters wanted to eliminate all discrimination and asked their employees and physicians to "work together for equal opportunities for men and women of all races."[67]

Pittsburgh: "Reaching Out to the Sick"

In some northern cities, including Pittsburgh, blacks comprised a smaller percentage of the population than in other cities, but neighborhoods were still mainly segregated.[68] In 1961, the Pittsburgh Catholic Interracial Council and Urban League undertook a study of the status of blacks in medicine in their city and found one black physician per 4,200 black citizens, with only thirty-six black physicians practicing in the metropolitan area. There was no municipal hospital and no all-black hospital. Indigent patients received care in voluntary hospital clinics, University of Pittsburgh clinics, and the Veterans Administration Hospital. While discrimination persisted in all the local hospitals, few administrators officially admitted its existence.[69] One who eventually would was Sister Ferdinand Clark, RSM, at Mercy Hospital.

Mercy was located in the heart of downtown, surrounded by low-income families, mainly blacks who had migrated to Pittsburgh after World War II. Many lived in the nearby Hill District. In the early 1960s, as the white middle class fled to the suburbs, the Sisters of Mercy, as we have seen, chose to stay. In 1964, they were turned down for a government grant to improve services to the Hill District, in large part because a powerful coalition of black citizens in the neighborhood opposed it. Sister Ferdinand, Mercy's administrator, quoted one of them: "You have treated us at Mercy. But you have never accepted us."[70]

There was considerable evidence of the truth of this charge. In 1946, the *Pittsburgh Courier*, a prominent black newspaper, reported stories of segregation from Pittsburgh Coal Company miners who were placed in a partitioned ward at Mercy, with whites on one side and blacks on the other. If white miners needed another bed on the ward, blacks were transferred to a separate convalescent area. Nurses (all white) were charged with ignoring blacks' needs. Other charges included segregation of black women patients and the lack of black doctors on the medical staff and of black nursing students in the training school. The sisters countered that blacks would be accepted to the school but that none had met the admissions criteria. Complicating the situation was a refusal by the sister administrator to publicly respond to the *Pittsburgh Courier* charges. Whether this specific situation influenced the Pittsburgh Coal Company is unclear, but in 1949 it ended its long association with Mercy and sought hospital services closer to the sites where injuries occurred.[71]

By 1960, Mercy had black pharmacy interns apprenticing with Sister Gonzales Duffy, RSM, the hospital's chief pharmacist, as they worked toward master's degrees in hospital pharmacy. The sisters eventually hired one of these interns. Still, in 1963 the Urban League reported a lack of full integration in all Pittsburgh hospitals, mainly in the area of semi-private rooms.

Although Mercy Hospital had black residents and interns, it still had no black physicians on staff.[72]

When the federal grant did not come through for Mercy's proposed expansion in 1964, the local community's poor opinion of the hospital shocked the Sisters of Mercy. Sister Ferdinand and Mercy's board of trustees developed a Human Relations Committee to review all complaints of racial discrimination and organized a Neighborhood Advisory Committee on Health Care, with representation from upper-, middle-, and lower-income residents in the area. Both committees held regular joint meetings so that the hospital could learn, at the grass-roots level, what residents wanted in terms of health care. These efforts did not go unchallenged, as some black neighborhood residents tried to resign, charging that Mercy Hospital was not training black staff for advancement and not recognizing the Neighborhood Advisory Committee's autonomy in operations. Their resignations were unanimously rejected, and Mercy worked on the areas of concern. Eventually a Neighborhood Advisory Committee member served on Mercy's board of trustees.[73]

The sisters themselves began attending community meetings in the Hill District, where at times the local residents screamed complaints at them. Unrest continued, with especially violent disturbances after the death of Martin Luther King Jr. in 1968. Because of Mercy Hospital's close proximity to the violence, emergency personnel took the injured there. Afterward the hospital instituted human relations seminars for all staff members to ensure they understood the social implications of Pittsburgh's racial problem. Outside experts conducted seminars on racial attitudes. Some sisters began serving on committees with the Urban League, the NAACP, the Mayor's Committee on Human Resources, and the Model Cities Program. Many attended nightly meetings of civil rights and community action groups, and they supported black arts festivals and established a black history library.[74]

Other efforts included providing scholarships for black students to the School of Nursing, training black students at Mercy for x-ray technology and medical photography, holding health career–training programs in cooperation with the local Office of Economic Opportunity, and conducting programs for alcoholism treatment. The hospital undertook a special advertising campaign to recruit black nurses from the South, brought one black doctor and one black dentist onto the hospital staff, and established a relationship with Meharry Medical College in Tennessee, a historically black medical school, to obtain interns. Mercy also recruited health care expediters from the Hill District to assist residents in obtaining health care. In 1969 the sisters opened a satellite clinic in the Hill District and followed this with two other neigh-borhood clinics, one for men in need and the other for elderly residents in a city-owned apartment complex. They set up the first Caremobile in Allegh-eny County, a traveling clinic staffed by a physician, nurse, social worker, and health care expediter. After breaking ground in 1968, Mercy followed an early trend by opening Mercy Health Center in 1970, which the Hospital Planning Association quickly approved. This was an ambulatory care facility with thirty-three examining rooms, multiple specialties, and ancillary ser-vices. In its first year, visits to Mercy Health Center totaled 26,831.[75]

When Sister Ferdinand retired as administrator in 1978, she considered her work to achieve adequate health care for blacks to have taught her one of the most meaningful and enduring lessons she had learned. "Inadequate health care only compounds the evils of poor housing and high unemploy-ment," she concluded. "Combined, these factors deny all minorities the right-ful place in society." In the mid 1970s, the Sisters of Mercy as a congregation conducted a social audit, asking members in all its institutions to concentrate on the dignity of the individual. At the hospital, this mandate included the public, vendors, employees, visitors, and most important, patients. By then, Mercy Hospital was more than an acute care institution; it had become deeply involved with the community it served. As Sister Ferdinand stated, the sis-ters "reach[ed] out to the sick, rather than waiting for them to come to us."[76]

"Good Business for Selma": The Civil Rights Movement

As in the rest of the segregated South, in Alabama blacks could not work in or be treated in white hospitals until the 1960s. Tuskegee Institute opened the first hospital and nurse training school in the state in 1892, which soon became a center for training black nurses and physicians. During the first half of the twentieth century, as a result of exclusion and discrimination else-where, southern black leaders worked with northern philanthropists such as the Rosenwald Fund and religious groups such as the Catholic Church to develop their own hospitals. More than twenty-five community-supported black hospitals were established in Alabama, including Good Samaritan Hos-pital in Selma, opened by the Sisters of Saint Joseph from Rochester, New York, in 1944.[77]

The Sisters of Saint Joseph (SSJs) were established as a white religious order in the mid-seventeenth century in France. After coming to Carondelet, Missouri, in 1836, they expanded to Canandaigua, New York, in 1854. The SSJs began their hospital ministry in 1908 when they opened a facility in

Elmira, New York. In Selma, the SSJs operated their hospital as a black institution within a legal system of segregation. They did not agree with the existing system, but they worked within it. Their efforts evolved over time to promote the economic and social development of blacks in the health professions. Since the 1940s, approximately a hundred sisters from Rochester have gone to Selma, and a third were nurses.[78] The others were teachers, community liaisons, and social workers. In providing a new hospital with up-to-date equipment and facilities, the sisters could offer black patients needed services.

Selma is the county seat and major town of Dallas County, and its racially exclusive policies necessitated separate facilities for blacks and whites in all areas of life. In 1944, Father Francis Casey, SSE, head of the Edmundite Mission in Selma, purchased Good Samaritan Hospital from the white physicians who had been operating it for black patients. Father Casey intended to staff it with the SSJs from Rochester who had come in 1940 when he appealed nationally for a religious congregation of women to help the priests of Saint Edmund in the mission for blacks. At that time, the sisters worked within the Catholic tradition of evangelization. In Selma, they at first visited the sick and poor, established a school for blacks, distributed clothing, and supervised recreations of the old and young.[79]

Sister Anastasia McCormack, SSJ, one of the first sisters to arrive in 1940, brought to Father Casey's attention the need of Selma's elderly population for a refuge for the dying; the result was the founding of Holy Infant Inn. When in 1944 Father Casey purchased Good Samaritan, Holy Infant Inn became part of that mission. Originally established as Baptist Good Samaritan Hospital in 1922 by local white doctors who also had founded Selma Baptist Hospital, Good Samaritan was intended to be a "separate but equal" facility for black patients. Physicians took over the administration from the Baptists in 1937 when the hospital was struggling during the Great Depression. To buy the deteriorating building in 1944, the Edmundites borrowed more than $80,000 dollars and also appealed to northern Catholics for support.[80]

Racial discrimination in Selma prevented most whites from supporting black hospitals. In his letter to Mother Rose Miriam Smyth, SSJ, requesting the sisters' services, Father Casey was straightforward in presenting the challenges.[81] Despite public declarations of equality, the institution was in fact separate and unequal. Nurses and patients had endured dangers and harsh working conditions. There were no laundry facilities, and open fireplaces burning wood or coal provided the only heat. There was a scarcity of toilets and bath facilities, no hot water tanks, and so few eating utensils that patients had to eat with their fingers. Mattresses were infested with vermin and bed linen was minimal. Personnel worked twelve hours a day, seven days a week for a weekly salary of only three dollars.[82]

Whites often judged black nurses to be deficient in skill and training, Darlene Clark Hine notes, despite evidence to the contrary.[83] Father Casey may have held this belief, for he stated that the physicians could not find qualified black registered nurses to supervise the institution. Casey and the doctors agreed that neither patients nor doctors benefited from the current arrangement, and that expert supervision was needed to remedy the situation. Father Casey's main interest, he admitted, was spiritual, but he also was concerned about the material good of the black population.[84] The assignment to Selma met Mother Rose Miriam's goal to establish a mission for blacks, and she sent the needed nurses.

The priests owned the hospital and obtained financial support through donations, while the sisters supervised it on salaries that covered only their living expenses. The first administrator was Sister Louis Bertrand Dixon, SSJ, who served from 1945 to 1964. She had graduated from Saint Joseph Hospital School of Nursing in Elmira, New York, in 1925 and earned her bachelor of science degree in nursing education at the Catholic University of America in Washington, D.C., in 1936. During her twenty-year tenure, she oversaw the hospital's growth from a small frame house, through a new brick extension in 1947, a second in 1957 that included an extended care facility, to a modern four-story structure in 1964 with 111 beds, 40 of which were reserved for the elderly. By then, Good Samaritan was the only hospital for blacks within a six-county area.[85]

Burns were common, and eventually the nuns established a separate area for burn care. One young girl who had fallen into the open fireplace in her home said, "The fire jumped on me." A sister nurse noted that the girl joined "the ranks of those poor, deformed, sad-eyed children" who spent months at Good Samaritan. Some came to the hospital "with arms or legs burned off and faces horribly burned." The hospital also admitted children with birth defects, including cleft lip, cleft palate, and clubfoot.[86]

The SSJs' convent, hospital, and school were located in Selma's black community, and the nurses encountered many patients whose lives were affected by poverty and racism. Of an eighteen-year-old with tuberculosis of the spine who weighed only seventy pounds and was in a heavy body cast, a sister noted: "She is poor. Her mother couldn't care for her. Who would care for an advanced T.B. for nothing?" Of another patient who required a reduction of a dislocated arm and planned to work in the summer to pay the hospital bill, the sister wrote: "The parents are separated, therefore the burden of support rests on the mother," but for black women, "it is next to impossible to earn more than a bare living in the South."[87] Good Samaritan Hospital also frequently received patients with injuries caused from beatings by the Ku Klux Klan.

Good Samaritan Hospital School of Practical Nursing

As more patients came to the hospital, a nursing shortage developed. To obtain trained nurses, Sister Louis Bertrand established Alabama's first school of practical nursing in 1950. Whereas most Catholic nursing orders maintained registered nursing schools for whites, the Good Samaritan Hospital program was for black students in practical nursing, although the sisters advertised it as open to everyone regardless of race, color, or creed. In establishing a practical school instead of a program for registered nurses, the nuns followed the philosophy of Booker T. Washington, founder of Alabama's Tuskegee Institute in 1881, who had encouraged blacks to focus on the practical issues of life, on things that needed to be done immediately. Although criticized then and since for encouraging blacks to forgo a broad education, he argued that blacks should first establish a practical base for advancement.[88] To him, social uplift strategies were key to obtaining racial equality. Thus the sisters' school brochure stated as an objective: "To prepare professional women, equipped physically, intellectually and spiritually, to provide self-satisfaction and community welfare."[89] One news release proudly noted that the wages of the thirty-five graduates of the School of Practical Nursing currently employed at Good Samaritan Hospital totaled more than $80,000, which boosted Selma's economy.[90]

The sisters worked predominantly with poor blacks in Selma and so designed a program that would enable students to enhance their employability and earning power in a relatively short time. The students and graduates also helped staff the growing hospital. Most were non-Catholic, although the sisters reported an average of four or five converts a year. The religious mission of the hospital was also reflected in its School of Nursing brochure, which promised that well-qualified applicants, "under the guidance of Religion and Catholic Philosophy," would "develop a Christ-like spirit toward the sick." Applicants had to have finished at least eight years of grammar school, with preference given to those who had completed high school. Each class comprised twenty to forty students; with no living facilities provided, those who were not from Selma boarded with local black families. They had their classes in the nursing home lounge and Saint Elizabeth's Parish Hall until a remodeled classroom space opened on the second floor of the hospital.[91]

The sisters taught the classes, with physicians providing guest lectures. Students received one year of theory and practice in medical, surgical, pediatric, and geriatric nursing. Sister Mary Christopher Kuchman, SSJ, broke the color barrier when she took the students to a white hospital in Montgomery so they could have obstetric clinical experience. By doing so, she was able to get the school accredited with the state. Other courses included anatomy and physiology, bacteriology, sociology, religion, and ethics. By 1966, the Good Samaritan School of Practical Nursing had graduated more than three hundred students, eight of whom were men. Graduates readily secured employment in hospitals throughout the South. Many of these nurses went on to get advanced degrees, while others stayed to work at Good Samaritan.[92]

Etta Perkins, one of the early graduates, became a registered nurse and taught in the sisters' nursing program. In June 1981 at the Thirty-fifth Annual Convention of the Licensed Practical Nurses Association of Alabama, she recalled that in the 1940s, "there was no place for a black girl in our area to go for training." When Sister Louis Bertrand set up Good Samaritan's school, it "opened the doors for us all."[93] The keynote speaker at that convention was Reverend William R. Wrench, a black registered nurse anesthetist who was then director of anesthesia at Good Samaritan Hospital. Several Good Samaritan alumni received awards. Thus the nuns' strategies paid off for many of their students, who joined the developing black professional class.[94]

When Good Samaritan became a Catholic hospital, white physicians provided the health care, led by a medical missionary, Dr. Isabell M. Dumont from Germany and Joan Mulder, a laboratory and x-ray technician. Black physicians did not predominate, because most were driven to locate in large cities, where the largest black clientele resided. In 1944, fifteen white, Protestant doctors comprised the staff of Good Samaritan Hospital. Five years later, seven lay registered nurses, including one man and three graduates from the sister's hospital in Elmira, New York, were working in the hospital. In a newsletter to potential donors, a priest noted that 698 baptisms had occurred in Selma, 210 of them administered to dying infants or during death-bed conversions, revealing the importance of the hospital in this mission activity.[95]

The women's congregation kept statistics not only of numbers but also of the race and religion of its workers. By 1958 twenty-two full- or part-time Protestant physicians were employed, only two of whom were black. By contrast, the majority of the personnel were Protestant blacks who worked under the sisters' supervision. The nuns, too, recorded their successes in baptisms: in 1959, forty-one infants, fifteen children, eight adults, and ten stillborn infants.[96] Good Samaritan Hospital became one of the largest employers in Selma, with 110 full-time and 10 part-time workers. During the twelve-month period ending June 30, 1964, its employees collectively earned more than $183,000. That year, 2,189 patients were admitted, 256 babies were born, and 1,479 emergency treatments were performed.[97]

Several SSJs reflected on their experiences as tension built in Selma in the early 1960s. Because they worked with blacks, many of Selma's white population considered the SSJs "black" by association. They were often designated the "black sisters" to distinguish them from the Sisters of Mercy, the "white sisters" who taught Selma's white children—although the Sisters of Mercy wore black habits and the SSJs wore white ones. The SSJs interpreted their identification with blacks as evidence of success in their mission. But in the minds of some white Selmians, the sisters' association with blacks made them outcasts, and the nuns often were subjected to derision.[98] Sister Josepha Twomey, SSJ, a teacher, recalled the fear she felt when crossing a street as a car came up behind her. She walked faster, and as the white driver gunned the engines and sped past, he shouted, "Nigger lover!" She was trembling as she reached the other side of the street. Sister Mary Paul Geck, SSJ, superior of the sisters in Selma, recalled that the sisters had three strikes against them: they were white, Catholic, and worked with blacks.[99]

The SSJs learned to manipulate the ambiguity of their racial position, Koehlinger effectively argues, sometimes claiming a "black" identity when they thought it would help their black neighbors, and other times strategically maintaining their whiteness, such as when acting as professional nurses and teachers.[100] The designation "black sister," however, did not mean that racial tensions were absent from Good Samaritan Hospital. In June 1960, for instance, hospital employees requested a meeting with Sister Louis Bertrand to ask for a raise and cab fare for those on the evening shift. Significantly, they asked to be addressed as "Mr., Mrs., or Miss."[101]

The sisters' racial ambiguity confounded the binary classification of black and white and challenged neat categorizations of segregation.[102] This was apparent in the sisters' participation in the voting rights movement in Selma. Blacks made up almost half Selma's population, but only 2 percent were registered voters. As the sisters observed the discrimination to which blacks were subjected, they began advocating for voting rights in subtle ways.

For example, they boycotted Selma's grocery stores that catered only to whites, buying groceries in Montgomery, fifty miles away; and they stood in "Colored Only" lines to show their support for blacks. On one occasion, when Sisters Josepha, Barbara Lum, SSJ, and Loretta Poole, SSJ, stopped at a local ice cream parlor and witnessed blacks, money in hand, being refused service, they left without getting served themselves.[103] Sister Mary Paul wrote to friends: "We most definitely are NOT neutral. For all practical purposes, we are 'Negroes' living in a Negro community. Actually we do not think in terms of color. Nor do the children or our people think of us that way."[104]

Since the late 1950s, individual leaders and the Dallas County Voters League (DCVL) had attempted to register black citizens to vote, but the White Citizens' Council and the Ku Klux Klan had kept blacks from registering and voting through discrimination and intimidation tactics. Then in 1963, in cooperation with the DCVL, the Student Nonviolent Coordinating Committee (SNCC), a principal organization of the civil rights movement, began organizing meetings and voter registrations in Selma and surrounding counties. The sisters grew increasingly sorrowful and angry over the cruelty they witnessed during these days. Sister Barbara had joined the hospital nursing staff in 1959 after working at the nuns' hospital in Elmira, New York, and taught in the practical nursing program in the 1960s. In a letter to her parents in May 1963, she wrote that several of the Good Samaritan nurses attended a meeting on voting registration in the Baptist church next door to the convent. She was very distressed by the nurses' reports that Sheriff Jim Clark came to the meeting and stood in the back of the church, because whites from several counties around Selma had often formed posses under Clark and followed African Americans to and from their meetings.[105] The sisters were horrified by the harassment of the black nurses at Good Samaritan Hospital, particularly after the bombing of the Sixteenth Street Baptist Church in Birmingham on September 15, 1963, that killed four young girls attending Sunday school. The violence set off sympathy sit-ins, picketing, and parading in the streets of Selma. In response, sheriff's deputies and highway patrolmen wearing steel helmets were very much in evidence, often arresting up to ninety black people a day, even though whites were behind most of the violence. When Sister Barbara took some of the nursing school's forty new students to the Health Department for a public health nursing experience, the media and the police showed up. Police cars followed some of the students home, mistaking them for voting protestors. That same month, Etta Perkins, an African American nurse at Good Samaritan Hospital, stood in line at the courthouse every day for two weeks to register to vote. Another black nurse was arrested for stopping to talk to a protester.[106]

By 1964, with the racial situation more intense, the sisters' stories emphasized their identification with the plight of their black neighbors. In July, seventy people, mostly teenagers, were arrested. Not long afterward, the nuns tried to visit a group of black students who had been jailed. On that occasion, their white skins brought them no privileges. Rather, the sisters saw hatred in the guards' eyes as they pointed guns at them. The sisters had brought food for the students, and a sister nurse wanted to make sure they were all right, but the guards refused them admittance.[107] On another occasion, one of their eighth-grade students had been arrested on the streets of Selma and detained several days for refusing to call a black woman by her first name; rather, she used "Mrs."[108]

On February 18, 1965, a trooper shot a young, unarmed civil rights protestor, Jimmie Lee Jackson, as he shielded his mother in a café, where they had fled after being attacked by troopers during a demonstration in nearby Marion. He was taken to Good Samaritan, where he died a week later. Sister Barbara cared for Jackson and, with tears welling in her eyes, she recalled him saying, "Don't you think this is a high price for freedom?"[109]

Bloody Sunday, March 7, 1965

The death of Jackson and the demonstrators' hopes of bringing attention to civil rights violations led to plans for a march on March 7, 1965, which came to be labeled Bloody Sunday. Good Samaritan Hospital became the primary facility for those injured when law enforcement officers attacked six hundred marchers as they tried to cross the Edmund Pettus Bridge for the fifty-two-mile march to Montgomery. Television cameras captured Sheriff Clark's lawmen tear-gassing, clubbing, spitting on, whipping, and jeering at the demonstrators, while others trampled on the marchers with horses as they drove them back into Selma.

Mobile's archbishop Thomas Toolen had forbidden the priests and nuns in his diocese to march, threatening to send back to their home state anyone who did so—a classic example of the use of ecclesiastical authority.[110] On the morning of March 7, the sisters were either at the hospital working their usual shifts or in Saint Elizabeth's convent. Sister Barbara had gone to the hospital to prepare a first-aid kit. She recalled her naiveté in fixing up a small box with Band-Aids, skin creams, and the like. No one expected violence, even though the sister nurses had cared for patients injured by whites in the past.[111]

Soon after they heard the news broadcast, the sisters received a phone call from Good Samaritan administrator Sister Michael Ann Hanley, SSJ, to send all the nurses immediately to the hospital. (Sister Michael Ann had succeeded Sister Louis Bertrand the previous year.) A few minutes later, a call came for all the sisters to hurry over. The hospital, staffed by 150 employees, 90 percent of whom were black, had a three-bed emergency room. Sisters Mary Paul and Mary Weaver, SSJ, elementary school teachers at Saint Elizabeth School that the SSJs ran for black children, sat at the admissions desk and processed incoming patients. They sent people overcome with tear gas to the dining room and the more seriously injured to the emergency room, where sister nurses Barbara and Saint Joseph Creighton, SSJ, cared for them, including John Lewis, the SNCC chair. Sister Liguori Dunlea, SSJ, another nurse, led those who were discharged to the extended care facility in the hospital and contacted relatives and friends for them. Sisters Margaret Isabelle Tracy, SSJ, and Mary Christopher cared for others in the hospital's dining room, now a second emergency room. Sister Josepha, a teacher, worked in the central supply room and helped Sisters Mary Weaver and Bernice Quinn, SSJ, transport people to x-ray and give spiritual and emotional support to the patients and their relatives.[112]

Men, women, boys, and girls came pouring into the hospital. Both white and black physicians came to help, as well as other off-duty nurses and personnel, including nurse Perkins and assistant administrator John Crear. Injuries included severe head lacerations, cuts and bruises, and limbs fractured by trampling horses. All the injured suffered from tear gas that had soaked their clothing; before long, in the enclosed rooms of the hospital, the nurses and other workers felt the effects as well. "I can still smell that smell," recalled Sister Barbara. "Everybody suffered from it. It's very pungent." Patients continued to arrive throughout the afternoon, and the workers tended more than a hundred people; they admitted to the hospital fifteen with head injuries and fractures.[113]

The televised images sickened and outraged people throughout the country. Following a call by Dr. Martin Luther King Jr., political and religious leaders and other sympathizers, including Catholic sisters, congregated in Selma with King to show their solidarity with the marchers. Although the SSJs could not march, they offered their hospital and convent as meeting and resting places for demonstrators from all across the country. In addition to 145 laypersons, the roster for visitors at Good Samaritan Hospital contained the names of five monsignors, 135 priests, thirty Protestant ministers, four rabbis, and two members of the U.S. Air Force. They came from twenty-six states, the District of Columbia, Canada, and Germany. Dr. King visited the hospital, as well, and other demonstrators stayed in the homes of Selma's black citizens (see figure 9).[114]

Father Maurice Ouellet, SSE, opened the parish house to civil rights workers as their base, an act that would contribute to his later expulsion from the diocese by his archbishop. This demonstrated the division among Catholics, many of whom believed that politics and religion should be separate. But Sister Barbara remembered: "It felt wonderful to have them coming. . . . I felt very proud to be a sister."[115]

Since male dominance still defined the Catholic Church, the archbishop allowed priests to attend civil rights meetings but forbade nuns to do so. Not wanting to directly challenge their superior, the sisters complied, yet they

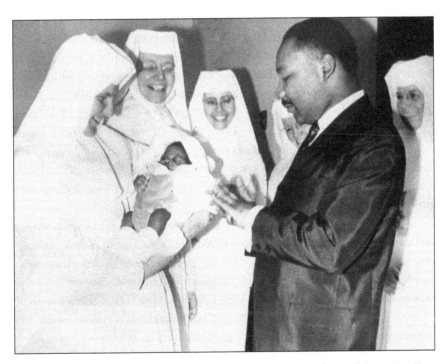

Figure 9   Dr. Martin Luther King Jr. with Sisters of Saint Joseph, Good Samaritan Hospital, Selma, Alabama, 1965. *From left*: Sisters Josepha Twomey, Dorothy Quinn, Mary Weaver, Margaret Isabel Tracy, and Mary Paul Geck. The baby, Synethia Perkins, was born at Good Samaritan on Dr. King's birthday.

Courtesy Society of Saint Edmund Archives, Saint Michael's College, Colchester, Vermont.

found creative ways to stretch the boundaries of Church discipline. When a noted civil rights figure and author, James Baldwin, spoke at the Baptist church next door to the convent, the sisters took turns standing on a convent radiator to hear his faint voice.[116] By engaging in this covert act of passive resistance, they found a measure of independence without having to wear the prickly cloaks of spiritual revolutionaries.

In the sisters' view, their hospital work was a form of "bearing witness," or of willingness to speak out against abuses, which was a new language nuns employed at the time to justify their actions in support of the civil rights movement. As one nursing sister recalled: "Little did we realize the morning of Monday, March 8, that our exhausting labors in 'bearing witness to Christ' were just beginning and would continue without respite for the month, and even beyond."[117]

Some clergy and laity attempted to thwart the demonstrators' actions, including Selma's mayor Joe Smitherman and Sheriff Clark. Archbishop Toolen saw the demonstrations, and particularly Dr. King, as divisive. Toolen was concerned about Ku Klux Klan reprisals against the area's Catholics, and he also feared that, if the clergy incited the local people, it would affect Selma's white Catholics' financial support of church programs, which was crucial for their success.[118] In his view, the demonstrations were "not helping things at all. . . . There are crazy people on both sides. As good citizens we should try to control them." The place of sisters and priests was "at home doing God's work."[119] Despite Toolen's disapproval, Catholic clergy and sisters from other parts of the United States converged on his diocese. Although it was customary for visiting priests and sisters to defer to the local bishop, this group did not.

The SSJs were familiar with white supremacy, and they prepared for the inevitable arrival of violence as more demonstrators came to Selma. As they readied themselves to care for the injured, they watched apprehensively as fifty-four priests and nuns from the Midwest, including six sisters from the Lorettos, the Sisters of the Blessed Virgin Mary, the Sisters of Saint Joseph of Carondelet, and the Franciscan Sisters of Mary chartered a plane and arrived in Selma on March 10. Two of them were black nurses. Most religious nursing orders were racially segregated and thus discriminatory regarding who could be admitted to their congregations and where they could live or work. One of the nurses on the plane was Sister Ann Benedict, CSJ, from Saint Joseph's Hospital in Kansas City, the first black woman to enter the Sisters of Saint Joseph of Carondelet. The other nurse was Sister Mary Antona Ebo, FSM, one of the first black members of the Franciscan Sisters of Mary. Although she had been accepted into the congregation, she still felt like an outsider, having gone through a segregated novitiate program in order to take her vows. She also had graduated from one of the few nurse training schools for blacks in St. Louis. After graduation, her work assignment included the "blacks only" part of Saint Mary's Infirmary in St. Louis. At the time of the march, Sister Mary Antona was working as a medical librarian at Saint Mary's.[120] Still, racial and religious walls were crumbling.

King was impressed with the massive display of religious leaders working and protesting together. Although the mayor and police halted the protesters less than a block from where they started out, eventually Dr. King led marchers to Montgomery on March 21, 1965. Congress enacted the Voting Rights Act, signed by President Lyndon Johnson, on August 6, 1965.

The Closing of Good Samaritan

The fate of Good Samaritan Hospital illustrates the general trend among most historically black hospitals. After President Johnson signed Medicare and Medicaid into law in 1965, Sister Michael Ann announced that Good Samaritan Hospital had been certified and approved as a provider of hospital services to Medicare patients. The sisters wasted no time readying the hospital to meet the required standards and helping their senior citizens fill out their applications for the new program.[121] By then the hospital had expanded to include a maternity ward, a pediatrics unit, a forty-one-bed medical-surgical area on the third floor, three new operating rooms, a recovery room, and air conditioning. In the 1960s, new interventions were developing for cardiac arrhythmias, and Good Samaritan personnel kept up to date by ordering special equipment for use in cardiac emergencies. Sisters supervised in-service training sessions while other nurses attended coronary care institutes and emergency-room seminars.[122]

Hospitals receiving federal funds had to comply with the Civil Rights Act of 1964 and could not discriminate in admissions. While Medicare and Medicaid payments helped Good Samaritan's finances at first, a gradual exodus of white doctors and their black patients to newer facilities with specialty units occurred. In 1970, citing rising costs and scarcity of qualified faculty members, the governing board of Good Samaritan Hospital announced that the School of Practical Nursing would close.[123] In addition, vocational and trade schools in Selma and surrounding community colleges were providing similar services.

In December 1971 the General Council of the Sisters of Saint Joseph in Rochester met with regional coordinators and nursing sisters to discuss worsening conditions at Good Samaritan, including diminishing physician support. According to the sisters, when a new medical center had opened in Selma the previous year in conjunction with the physician-owned Baptist Hospital, physicians began referring patients there because of the center's specialized services such as cardiac care units. Good Samaritan leaders tried to recruit black physicians and doctors from a nearby U.S. Air Force base, with no success. Consequently, finances were precarious. Registered nurses were leaving, and nationwide efforts to recruit replacements were failing. On December 21, 1971, SSJ council members finalized the decision to withdraw from Good Samaritan Hospital and Nursing Home.[124]

When the SSJs pulled out in 1972, black leaders became more involved in the hospital; John Crear became administrator and Dr. Charles Lett the medical chief of staff. The hospital rebounded strongly, securing a grant for research on rural health in Dallas and surrounding counties. By 1981, Good Samaritan was providing a $1.5 million in free medical care and treating an average of five hundred charity cases a year. It had the highest percentage of Medicare and Medicaid patients of the twenty-three hospitals in southwest Alabama; but even when patients qualified for Medicaid, the hospital recouped only 85 percent of its costs.[125] Bed occupancy was down to 25 percent by 1983, and the increased overhead associated with paid staff made the financial problems overwhelming. The hospital had to close. The remaining elderly patients in the nursing home transferred to a facility in Montgomery.[126]

Many of the sisters who left Selma did not return to their traditional work in schools and hospitals but worked in new areas such as prisons, pastoral care, and clinics for the poor. Sister Catherine Teresa Martin, SSJ, used her business skills in Selma for another fourteen years. Notably, she worked with poor black women to put the Freedom Quilting Bee cooperative on firm ground; it is still active. Sister Mary Weaver, a teacher and social worker, also stayed in Selma and worked in schools, clinics, and government agencies to help people get loans, food, and assistance for heating bills in the winter. Some nurses continued to run the rural health clinics through the 1990s. Four SSJs engage in ministry in Alabama today.[127]

In summary, the sister nurses trained and worked side by side with the black nursing staff, and together they opened doors of acceptance and opportunity for Selma's black community. Since the SSJs were deeply embedded in a hierarchical and patriarchal church, however, they obeyed their archbishop's orders not to march or attend civil rights meetings in Selma in 1965, although they bristled at it. They searched for a middle ground between obedience and conscience. These sisters did not see themselves as powerless in combating racism. They had the support of their religious community, and the Catholic Church gave them legitimacy.[128] At the same time, their hospital in Alabama played an important role in the professional education and practice of black nurses, both women and men, at a time when their options were limited. Blacks obtained self-confidence and status that bolstered them in pursuing various social and civic opportunities. Indeed, the hospital's employment of a large number of blacks at decent wages gave them independence from Selma's dominant white establishment. Finally, as the sisters' identities merged with those of blacks and they received some of the same hate-filled attitudes and behaviors from whites, they better understood what Suellen Hoy meant by leading "a life in religion," a life of struggle, sacrifice, and empathy.[129]

Good Samaritan Hospital served black residents in Selma and the surrounding counties when other hospitals closed their doors to them. By the 1980s, however, when many black patients could routinely obtain care from specialists in any hospital, Good Samaritan was forced to close. Desegregation had proved fatal, as for other historically black hospitals.[130]

Conclusion

Throughout the nineteenth and twentieth centuries, race influenced all aspects of hospital cultures and operations across the country. In the 1950s, social and religious changes were destabilizing society, as well as Catholic and non-Catholic health care institutions. As cities experienced racial strife, religious congregations responded with mixed results. Racial barriers that divided Americans for many years were reinforced in Pittsburgh and in Chicago's Catholic hospitals until the 1960s. In Chicago, it required the action of civic and religious authorities to undo segregation. That white physicians did not want black patients provided a ready excuse for some sister administrators, who capitulated to business realities and sacrificed their Catholic values of treating everyone regardless of race, creed, or financial status.

With exceptions noted in this chapter, many Catholic hospitals, while continuing to provide needed services to the poor and indigent, generally fell behind when it came to race relations and integration practices. Although the Alexian Brothers distinguished themselves by admitting the first black male student nurse to their program, most Catholic schools of nursing were not much better than hospitals in their integration policies. Despite some sisters' and brothers' activism, many Catholic hospitals and religious communities maintained segregation, both in patient care and in training, just as religious orders themselves were typically discriminatory in admissions to their ranks.

Actions in those spheres were often rationalized as prudent, but in hindsight perhaps a more accurate term is "timid." Some Catholic hospital leaders, in their effort to maintain the racial status quo, missed an opportunity to speak out against racism. With Catholicism's history as a minority Christian religion in the United States, one might think that Catholics would have done more to champion the rights of other minorities. One could argue, however, that many Catholics were reticent to bring more public scorn on themselves by identifying strongly and openly with blacks.

Still, by the mid 1960s, however, many sisters and brothers were primed for the changes ushered in by Vatican II, with its emphasis on social justice and human dignity for all people. Now many were unambiguous in their opposition to racism. Their work with blacks put them in conflict with their superiors, other congregation members, and the laity over what was appropriate work for women and men dedicated to religious service. The Sisters of Mercy in Pittsburgh and Chicago took leadership roles in addressing the inequity of segregation in their inner cities, and they reached out effectively and compassionately in service to their neighboring communities. Furthermore, as black sisters of the Catholic Church, long perceived as a white institution, joined the civil rights struggle, they transformed themselves and the Church. After her march in Selma, Sister Mary Antona helped establish the National Black Sisters' Conference and later served as its president. In 1976, when she was named administrator of Saint Clare Hospital in Baraboo, Wisconsin, she became the first black woman religious to head a hospital.[131]

Chapter 5

Catholic Hospitals and the Federal Government

Consistent with their support of racial justice, Catholic hospital leaders eventually supported the right of all to affordable health care. In 1981, with competition growing between general and investor-owned hospitals, the U.S. Conference of Catholic Bishops (USCCB) called for a national health insurance program.[1] But this was a change in policy. Catholic and non-Catholic hospital leaders had traditionally resisted government intervention in their affairs, early on opposing a national health insurance program managed by the government. Over the last quarter of the twentieth century, however, Catholic health care leaders softened their stance as they extended their religious values in the area of universal health care, and they called for greater government intervention. They also added the prevention of abortion and reproductive services to their policy agenda. These events offer a lens through which to view the role Catholic hospitals have played in overall U.S. health policy, and how Catholic leaders have defined their roles in light of the larger society.

As early as the eighteenth century, Catholics in the United States endorsed separation of church and state, religious tolerance, and religious pluralism.[2] This separation, however, did not affect their engagement with the government over issues they deemed important. In 1909, Monsignor John Ryan, a priest on the faculty of Catholic University of America, strongly advocated a minimum wage that would help workers afford medical care. Ryan stated his claims in terms of human rights, which was exceptional for that day, and based on religious principles espoused in Pope Leo XIII's 1891 *Rerum Novarum* (Of

New Things), the Church's first social encyclical to address workers' rights. In succeeding years, popes broadened and refined those teachings, primarily through encyclical letters.[3]

During World War I, Catholics for the first time had the confidence to speak as an American body through the National Catholic War Council to assist servicemen and servicewomen, an organization that became the National Catholic Welfare Council after the war, later the National Catholic Welfare Conference. Catholics earlier had been active in municipal politics and building Catholic institutions such as schools and hospitals, as a group focusing on servicing their own members, who were primarily immigrants, but by the 1930s, they were ready to progress to the national arena.[4]

As the number of Catholic hospitals increased, their leaders recognized their potential for power in the policy arena. They consistently argued that voluntary hospitals should be equal partners with public or governmental institutions that were run by city, county, state, or federal governments. Using a rhetoric of service, they asserted that they were charitable institutions providing a community benefit.[5] But there lay the tension, as Catholic hospitals also were growing in technology and science and providing services for a fee.[6]

The Politicization of Catholic Hospitals

The Catholic Hospital Association (CHA) formed in 1915 to bring Catholic hospitals into compliance with the hospital standardization movement. While sisters, priests, and physicians played significant roles in hospitals, conservative bishops and priests prohibited nuns from being appointed presidents and other full-time officers. The CHA originated as the sisters' organization since they ran most of the Catholic hospitals, but their own congregations had rules that constricted their travel and attendance at meetings. Until the 1960s, priests held the highest leadership positions, although sisters could serve on executive boards, head committees, participate in conventions, make speeches on hospital policies, testify before Congress, and set standards for Catholic nursing education. Beginning in the 1930s the major hospital associations, including the CHA, became political lobbies at the state and national levels.[7]

Individual sister nurses such as Sister John Gabriel Ryan, SP, were foot soldiers in this movement. A member of the Sisters of Providence congregation in Seattle, Sister John Gabriel in the 1930s worked extensively with social and legislative issues as they related to hospitals and nursing. With a master's degree earned in 1937, she served as hospital consultant and directress of schools of nursing for the Sisters of Providence in the West and taught classes on nursing administration all over the country (see figure 10). She also was vice president of the Washington State Hospital Association, a councilor and member of the Legislative Committee for the Western Hospital Association, a member of the boards of directors of the Washington State Nurses Association and the *American Journal of Nursing*, vice president of the Seattle Hospital Council, and a member of the Advisory Committee of the Catholic Hospital Association. In 1935 she served on the advisory committee of the Hospital Board of the Committee on Economic Security in Washington, D.C. The author of five books on nursing, she was a member of the editorial staff of three national hospital journals.[8]

In 1935, Sister John Gabriel was awarded an honorary fellowship in the American College of Hospital Administrators (ACHA), formed independently

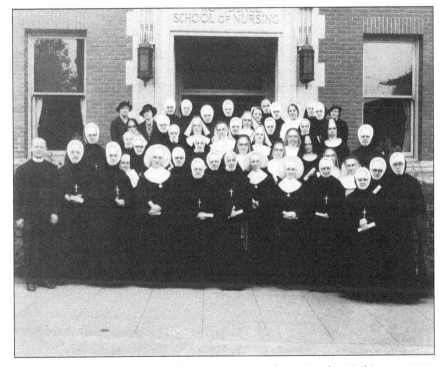

Figure 10 Class at the School of Nursing, Providence Seattle, Washington, 1935, probably taught by Sister John Gabriel, first row, far right.

HCA.D7.2, Providence Archives, Mother Joseph Province, Seattle, Washington.

of the American Hospital Association (AHA) in 1933 as a professional association for nonphysician and physician administrators. This organization
validated what Sister John Gabriel had been advocating for years: the need
for further education of hospital administrators, including her own sisters.
Malcolm MacEachern, director of the American College of Surgeon's Standardization Program, became an honorary charter fellow of the ACHA and
worked extensively with Sister John Gabriel in matters of hospital policy.
Sister John Gabriel drew greater attention for the new program of hospital
accreditation to Pacific Northwest hospitals and was a leader in preparing
sisters for nursing and administrative work. Her courses in hospital administration throughout the United States and Canada laid a basic foundation for
this field in nursing programs, and she tied her courses to colleges for credit
wherever she taught.[9]

The Great Depression created emergencies that caused a flood of legislation affecting all of U.S. society, including hospitals.[10] Besides collecting
fewer receipts, hospitals were providing more free meals to the unemployed.
As one sister lamented, society took it for granted that, because sisters managed Catholic hospitals, they were "miraculously sustained without mone-
tary assistance."[11] Voluntary hospitals also faced more competition from the
government. Between 1909 and 1932, hospitals grew six times as fast as the
general population. A quarter of the country's population was unemployed;
when these people got sick, they flocked to the institutions where they did
not have to pay. Thus, of the 776 general hospitals run by the government,
77.1 percent were occupied, compared to 55.9 percent of the 3,529 nongov-
ernmental general hospitals.[12] The shift to public institutions prompted voluntary hospitals' leaders to fight even greater government influence, and the
CHA increasingly worked to shape the public's perception of the voluntary
hospital, taking a leadership role in defining Catholic hospitals as charitable
institutions with a public mission and identity.[13]

As the poor economy and expanding demands for free care led hospital
associations and administrators to work together in the political arena, they
became avid proponents of the value of voluntary hospitals over government
provision. In 1932, for example, Dr. E. T. Olsen from Detroit spoke at the AHA
meeting: "At no time in the history of the American Hospital Association have
the hospitals been troubled by problems such as we have at the present time,
which threaten to break down our voluntary hospital system."[14] To expand
their influence on public policy, three national associations, the American
Hospital Association, Catholic Health Association, and Protestant Hospital

Association formed a joint committee that became an active political lobby, presenting a united front in debates over President Franklin Roosevelt's New Deal programs. The joint committee's principal aims were to ensure that voluntary hospitals were included in any federal legislation and that the dual system of government and voluntary institutions be preserved.[15] By the end of 1932, what Rosemary Stevens labels a "joint rhetoric of voluntarism" was in place; members of the joint committee testified at hearings on federal legislation that affected hospitals.[16] The CHA had an additional responsibility: to conform to the thought of the Catholic hierarchy in the United States. Thus it developed an affiliate relationship with the National Catholic Welfare Conference, the agency created by bishops to promote Catholic interests at the national level.[17]

A major aim of the CHA and other voluntary associations was to project a caring image that would allow them to receive nonpaying patients at the government's expense.[18] They were especially concerned over the growing veterans' hospital system and the increased competition it brought. Furthermore, participants in New Deal programs such as the Civil Works Administration received free or reimbursed medical care, and voluntary hospitals feared that they would go only to public hospitals. A delegate to the 1934 CHA convention explained that the country did "not need more public hospitals, but public help for the private hospital."[19] The joint committee saw no reason why its hospitals should not be included in legislation aimed at improving the health of the nation. While insisting that voluntary hospitals would continue to take on responsibility for charity patients, the joint committee pressed the government to help them pay for indigent care.[20]

The CHA, in particular, was outspoken on the question of who had responsibility for indigent patients. At its 1933 convention, members resolved that "this Association cannot and does not regard the indigent as the ward solely of the state and that it record its unwillingness to resign the valued privilege of caring for Christ's poor . . . into the hands solely of governmental agencies."[21] The CHA defined indigents as "wards of society," implying that they had a right to receive care from voluntary hospitals. While this stance left room for the role of religion in providing care for individuals and communities, it also provided the rationale for indigent patients in Catholic hospitals to be subsidized by the government. Resolutions asking for government aid were passed at the 1934 CHA convention, but money could be accepted under only one condition: "federal relief to hospitals does not mean federal control." Implicit in the CHA's resolution was the fear that the government might challenge hospital leaders' authority by becoming more involved in management issues. Eventually, the joint committee secured a ruling that allowed government employees to be admitted to voluntary hospitals with reimbursement from the federal government but without significant government regulation.[22]

The enactment of the National Reconstruction Administration (NRA), which established codes of fair practice for industrial and commercial industries, again galvanized the joint committee. In 1934, MacEachern asked Sister John Gabriel to speak before the American College of Surgeons Conference in Spokane, Washington, on the role of hospitals in President Roosevelt's recovery program. She stated her support for the New Deal, often using patriotic rhetoric—"to help our President realize his ambition" to forge the nation's economic recovery. Yet the federal NRA codes would regulate fair practices by establishing higher salaries and shorter working hours, which the already financially strapped hospitals could not afford. The codes also guaranteed employees the right of collective bargaining, to which Catholic hospitals objected—indeed, voluntary hospitals typically paid their employees less than prevailing wage rates. The voluntary associations asked for exemption from the codes.[23]

Sister John Gabriel also reminded the surgeons that her congregation's hospitals had already cut expenses and practiced strict economy except where patient welfare was concerned. "Their list of activities cannot be restricted without added cost of illness to the public, which the public cannot meet," she explained. They had shortened the hours of some personnel to allow more employees to work. The attorney for the NRA agreed with the joint committee's argument that voluntary hospitals were charitable organizations and did not come within the scope of the NRA—saving the voluntary hospitals large sums of money in payrolls.[24]

Sister John Gabriel laid out another argument: it was essential that voluntary hospitals, as not-for-profit institutions, continue to be recognized as tax-exempt facilities. She described how the joint committee worked to assure that no legislation impinged upon this right, securing a ruling from the Treasury Department that exempted hospitals from a 5 percent tax on dividends and securities they held in trust. She concluded: "The joint committee has seen the need of keeping a hospital representative in Washington to safeguard our policies and protect us in future hospital legislation—a wise and profitable [move] to which we should all lend our cooperation."[25] Agreements with the government brought five million Civil Works Administration patients to voluntary hospitals, and exemptions from the NRA saved the private institutions $20 million.[26]

The joint committee's success with the NRA was a stepping-stone toward lobbying nationally on other issues, and in the 1930s and 1940s it participated in nearly all legislation that affected hospitals. For example, it lobbied successfully in 1935 to get an exemption for charitable hospitals and their employees from the payment of Social Security. Hospital employees did not get Social Security benefits until the 1950s in some states, and their payment was not mandatory until 1983.[27]

Sister John Gabriel was active in these policy initiatives and in local, state, and national hospital and nursing associations. She contributed frequently to convention programs through papers and discussions, and she wrote extensively about the value of the voluntary hospital. She went to Washington, D.C, and to Olympia, Washington's capital, to speak on matters of policy in order to further desirable legislation or to oppose dangerous proposals.[28] For example, she was instrumental in helping to defeat a state senate bill that would have allowed the admission of chiropractors and osteopaths to hospital staffs; she considered these practitioners "dangerous cultists" who did "unlawful, inhuman things." When the bill was being discussed, she sat in the gallery and personally lobbied one of the senators. "This is not a denominational question," she argued later, "nor a political question, but a humane question concerned with suffering humanity which is looking to us for protection."[29] Some might call Sister John Gabriel's verbal attacks extreme, but none who knew her would dare to question her sincerity. And the presence of a nun in the gallery, wearing her traditional religious habit, was surely influential.

A justice of the Supreme Court of Washington State remarked to another sister: "She took a man's name in religion, and I said of her that she was the ablest man in Olympia."[30] Her masculine name helped Sister John Gabriel transcend female stereotyping, which minimized gender limitations, an advantage in the male-dominated realm of public policy.[31] The battles she chose to fight were related to her special interests: hospitals and the nursing profession. To achieve her aims, she aligned herself with the men who wielded the greatest power, particularly those who led hospital associations. Sister John Gabriel retired in 1938.

The Problem of Taxes

Charitable hospitals in many states had received some form of local tax relief since 1900, and their leaders monitored any legislation that proposed changes.[32] Catholic hospitals, like other voluntary institutions, were legally classified as charitable facilities, making them exempt from income taxation on the grounds that any net income would be put back into the hospital for services to the public and expansion of facilities. In 1942, however, the tax advisor to the U.S. secretary of the treasury recommended that charitable or educational institutions be subject to taxes on their income from trade or businesses not necessarily incident to their tax-exempt status. Furthermore, bequests for charitable purposes, until then deductible in estate taxes, would be limited to a percentage of the decedent's estate. In a letter to the chair of the House Ways and Means Committee, the National Catholic Welfare Conference protested that the legislation restricted charitable institutions' power to own property. At its 1942 convention, the CHA concurred: this proposal discriminated against charitable institutions, and if bequests were taxed, Catholic hospitals would be put at a distinct disadvantage.[33] Indeed, taxes would be so "dangerous" that they would destroy the hospitals and the great social services they rendered. The National Catholic Welfare Conference and CHA were successful in securing a continuation of the tax-exempt status of their institutions.[34]

National Health Legislation

In the development of federal legislation in the 1940s, only male Church leaders testified at committee hearings in Washington, D.C., and their most significant activity of the decade was to oppose a national health insurance program. Catholics had become involved in the progressive reform movement in the early twentieth century. In 1919, for example, Monsignor Ryan had authored the "Bishops' Program for Social Reconstruction," a blueprint for U.S. social and economic change. One of its provisions called for health insurance for the sick, unemployed, and aged. But the bishops believed that the best format was through employers; any contribution from the state should be temporary. Ideally, workers would be self-reliant enough to provide for their own needs, so "all forms of state insurance should be regarded as merely a lesser evil, and should be so organized and administered as to hasten the coming of the normal condition."[35]

During the Great Depression, as rising medical costs left the poor and working classes unable to pay for health care, access became a primary objective for policy makers.[36] As a result, health insurance, which had failed under the Progressives and socialists in the early twentieth century, was back on the national agenda. It followed upon the ineffectiveness of the Committee on the Costs of Medical Care (CCMC), established in 1927 to study the problem of high costs. The committee's final report in 1932 concluded that the costs of services were not adequately distributed, and it called for comprehensive medical care to be organized around hospitals. It also recommended that all basic public health services be extended to the entire population, and that medical costs be placed on a group payment basis through insurance. Influenced by the opposition of the American Medical Association (AMA), however, which did not want what it called "socialized medicine," President Roosevelt did not include health insurance in the Social Security Act of 1935, which did include funds for crippled children and maternal care. The only CCMC recommendation incorporated was federal grants to the states for public health programs. By the late 1930s, another CCMC recommendation, Blue Cross, a voluntary prepayment hospital insurance program, was growing nationally.[37]

In his State of the Union message in 1943, Roosevelt for the first time called for a social insurance system that would extend "from the cradle to the grave." Patterned after the Beveridge Report on social insurance that was presented to Great Britain's parliament in 1942, the Wagner-Murray-Dingell Bill for compulsory health insurance was introduced to the U.S. Congress in 1943.[38] It caused a storm of comment. Although organized labor backed it enthusiastically, representatives of physicians and the insurance industry vigorously opposed it. The CHA and other hospital associations also came out against the bill, fearing again that it would make patients wards of the state as opposed to wards of society and lead to the demise of the voluntary hospital.[39]

Using the language of charity, the CHA encouraged sisters and brothers to "jealously guard their right to give unremunerated care to the sick poor."[40] In condemning the monopoly of the government in caring for the sick and indigent, CHA leaders took their stand in the organization's official journal, *Hospital Progress*, in 1943, listing Catholic viewpoints toward the patient, disease, the physician, hospital service, and the government. The development of the national health program would not preserve the dignity of the patient, a key value of Catholic health care. Furthermore, a national program took social causes of disease such as unemployment and old age into account as significant factors in disease causation. Catholic views of illness had not yet endorsed this view, instead seeing illness in religious terms such as an opportunity for redemption; Catholic hospital leaders were not opposed to scientific progress in combating disease, but illness could be an opportunity for spiritual development. Regarding physicians, the doctor-patient relationship was of value; the Wagner bill would force doctors to become agents of the government. Hospital service had implications for the religious sisters and brothers who worked to render a "supernatural service": care of the sick and the indigent was a means for them to strive for spiritual perfection, which a government program could interrupt. Catholic hospital leaders decried the paternalism of the Wagner bill: by reducing a person's responsibility for his or her own health to legislative responsibility, the bill diminished human dignity. It was not only a "menace to the Catholic hospital but destructive of the Catholic attitude toward the patient." The CHA again insisted that the government should support both public and voluntary hospital services.[41]

The Wagner-Murray-Dingell bill not only advocated compulsory insurance but also spoke to the need for more hospital facilities. The joint committee of the three hospital associations sought to separate the two provisions. In 1944, before the bill died in committee, the joint committee evolved a plan for the cooperation of voluntary and government hospitals in meeting the health needs of the country.[42] Alphonse Schwitalla, the CHA president, and others on the joint committee for the first time sponsored a bill that they had helped develop, culminating in the Hill-Burton Act. The Hill-Burton bill was introduced to Congress in the spring of 1945; it provided federal grants to states for the construction of hospitals and health centers. In return, hospitals agreed to provide a reasonable amount of services to people unable to pay and to make their services available to all persons in the area.[43]

Schwitalla appeared before the Senate Committee on Education and Labor to support the Hill-Burton bill. He applauded its emphasis on state and local responsibility as they related to the federal role, and he particularly supported its provision for augmentation of existing facilities: new wings needed to be built, obsolete equipment replaced, and facilities brought into line with the newest scientific developments.[44] While the CHA supported the Hill-Burton bill, it suggested an important amendment that would weight the funds according to the extent of services given by public institutions and by voluntary hospitals. This would ensure that voluntary hospitals would get the utmost value from the program. Although unsuccessful in their amendment, the CHA and other members of the joint committee promoted the legislation. Significantly, the bill restricted the government's role to determining how funds would be distributed to states, which meant no federal strings attached. It also established the Federal Hospital Council composed of private citizens, which limited federal control. The Hill-Burton Act was signed into law in August 1946. Its passage represented a major contribution of the joint committee: it specified that funds would apply to both governmental and private not-for-profit hospitals, thereby recognizing the traditional dual hospital system in the United States.[45]

Planning for postwar hospital construction started before the end of World War II as hospital leaders anticipated that millions of returning veterans would need medical care. In addition, hospital admissions were rising due to dramatic advances in medical technology. By 1946, the Catholic health ministry was active in its building program. Schwitalla reported that of the 1,300 Catholic hospitals in the United States and Canada, 552 were reporting postwar expansion plans at an estimated cost of $150 million.[46] Under the Hill-Burton legislation, a formula that apportioned federal funds to states favored those with greater hospital deficiencies. Hospital beds in these states, especially in the South, increased significantly.[47] Within states, however, funds often went to middle-income communities, and inner-city hospitals had little support.[48] Still, the postwar years saw rapid expansion in the health care field. In 1945, there were 685 Catholic hospitals in the United States, with 87,171 beds. By 1950, these had increased to 739 hospitals and 96,349 beds. By 1960, there were more than 800 Catholic hospitals with 136,689 beds.[49]

Another issue surfaced in 1946 that threatened Catholic hospitals' independence. When the Social Security Act passed in 1935, it covered only workers in commerce and industry. In 1939, however, it expanded to cover dependents and survivors of such workers.[50] As this government program offered increased services, hospital leaders worried once again that the voluntary hospital would be reduced to the role of servant under the state. At the 1946 CHA meeting, the director of the Legal Department addressed the attendees, emphasizing Catholic hospitals' motivation of charity even in services rendered for which payment was made, and voicing concern that the state would not preserve Christian charity. Indeed, "experience alone could determine to what extent a truly Catholic hospital could maintain its identity under such a system." To that end, Catholic sisterhoods must work together and remain loyal and united with the CHA as their spokesperson.[51]

Of course, with priests at the head of the CHA, one might conclude that not only were sisters barred from filling organizational leadership roles, but also their voices were muted when it came to matters of governmental advocacy. Today we would label this gender discrimination. However, such practices reflected not only centuries of Catholic tradition, but also male-biased norms typical of the U.S. workplace of the 1940s. There were, to be sure, exceptions to such practices: Sister John Gabriel Ryan was a vocal advocate in hospital policy issues. Still, male leadership was deeply entrenched in health policy in market-related legislative initiatives.

In November 1945, Harry Truman became the first president to place the full weight of the office behind a plan for national health insurance. A revised Wagner-Murray-Dingell bill that proposed national health insurance under Social Security sparked debate over the next several years. The issue became enmeshed in the politics of the cold war, with opponents extolling capitalism as they linked the fight against socialized medicine to the crusade against communism. Roman Catholicism had opposed communism since *Rerum Novarum* condemned it in 1891. While the encyclical also criticized unfettered capitalism, it was the anticommunist language on which Catholics focused. After the war, as Catholic leaders again expressed their commitment to voluntary efforts, they did not embrace Monsignor Ryan's earlier view that everyone had a basic human right to health care, even through the government if necessary. Disagreements were minimal on this issue because Catholic leaders such as Monsignor John O'Grady of the National Conference of Catholic Charities expected private health insurance to expand quickly, offering coverage to many more people. Indeed, employer-provided insurance had grown during the war. Opponents succeeded in stalling the Wagner-Murray-Dingell bill in 1946.[52]

Truman made national health insurance a priority again in 1948, and hospitals and physicians across the country again opposed it. In her "Report of Management for 1948," the sister administrator at Mercy Hospital in Pittsburgh called the year one of "foreboding for private hospitals" due to "socialized medicine's" threat.[53] In 1949, fearing a loss of freedom for the voluntary hospitals, the CHA, National Catholic Welfare Conference, and Catholic Charities submitted their own plan to expand health insurance on a voluntary basis. They proposed that the federal government allocate $2.5 billion a year to the health care system, with $1.5 billion earmarked for tax credits for individuals to purchase health insurance through programs such as Blue Cross or Blue Shield. The rest of the funds were to be divided among grants to the states for indigent care; hospital construction and expansion, particularly in isolated and rural areas; medical and nursing education; dentistry; and research.[54]

In 1949, the AMA argued that compulsory sickness insurance would exclude the aged, those with chronic diseases, and underprivileged groups such as blacks and American Indians, who were not patients in most U.S. acute care hospitals. For these groups, special legislation would be required to provide facilities such as nursing homes and separate black hospitals.[55] The following year, black physicians criticized the AMA's separatist stance, and they particularly railed against Catholic hospitals. After the Chicago archdiocesan paper, the *New World*, published the Catholic plan, Dr. A. M. Mercer, president of the Cook County Physicians' Association, a black physicians' group, suggested that Catholics' opposition to a national health program was primarily to keep blacks out of their hospitals. He interpreted the Catholics' concern over government control as fear that the government would interfere with their hospitals' segregation practices. When Catholics said they wanted more federal grants for hospital construction, what they really wanted was to "take your money and mine while at the same time they bar us and our patients from their hospitals." Finally, aid to the state for the indigent to use voluntary hospitals would mean that blacks "would continue to be the human guinea pigs on which white doctors perfect their operative skill."[56]

Neither Truman's compulsory program nor the Catholic voluntary plan was successful.[57] Proponents of national health insurance abandoned their original proposals to concentrate on guaranteeing some form of coverage to the elderly. Whereas Presidents Truman, Eisenhower, and Kennedy introduced such legislation, it was not until 1965 during Lyndon Johnson's presidency, with a large Democratic majority in Congress, that the Kerr-Mills bill established Medicare and Medicaid to provide money for the care of the aged and the poor, respectively. Significantly, the provisions included, first, that private insurance companies chosen by the hospitals themselves would act as third parties for distributing funds. Second, reimbursements to hospitals would be based on costs rather than on set fee schedules. Thus, although the federal government made the payments, it did not regulate the prices or the billing procedures.[58]

Changes in Catholic Hospital Perspectives

Catholics' influence peaked after World War II when postwar affluence and the GI Bill helped increase Catholics' educational levels. Many men and women joined seminaries and convents and became priests and sisters. Nearly a hundred Catholics served in Congress, and others held other high political offices. The 1960s were the peak of Catholic prestige, especially with the election of John F. Kennedy as the first Catholic president. In 1963, Pope John XXIII included the right to health care in his list of individual human rights in the encyclical *Pacem in Terris* (Peace on Earth), and this time he proclaimed his message to the whole world rather than just to Catholics.[59] While Vatican II's documents did not give any specific instructions pertinent to health care services, they did provide general principles. For example, the Catholic social justice tradition was further rooted in *Gaudium et Spes* (Joy and Hope), or the "Pastoral Constitution on the Church in the Modern World," which emphasized that each person was worthy of dignity and respect and should be counted an equal member of society. Vatican II called on Church members to engage in and shape society rather than simply strengthening Catholic subcultures. Pope Paul VI followed in 1967 with the social encyclical *Populorum Progressio* (On the Development of Peoples), which inspired many men and women, laity and clerics, to dedicate themselves in service to the poor.[60] In 1971, in his document *Octogesimus Adveniens* (the Eightieth Anniversary), or "A Call to Action," Pope Paul broadened the definition of the poor to include the elderly and those disadvantaged by urbanization.[61] Thus after Vatican II the mission of Catholic hospitals encompassed more than caring for the sick—it also included social justice concerns and more aggressive advocacy for health care reform.

As Catholic influence over U.S. hospital policy was growing, "the most obvious phenomenon of hospital history since 1965 [was] the overwhelming force of national government policy," according to Stevens.[62] After the passage of Medicare and Medicaid increased federal involvement in health care, the new executive director of the CHA, Father Thomas F. Casey, SJ, noted that the association needed to expand its voice on public policy issues. Now, too, women religious were taking greater leadership roles in the public arena. In 1971, Sister Mary Maurita Sengelaub, RSM, became the first woman executive director of the CHA. A nurse and hospital administrator, she held a master's degree in hospital administration. Under her leadership, the association created the Office of Government Services in 1973 to advocate for CHA interests in health care legislation and regulation. This office moved to Washington, D.C., in 1976.[63]

By the 1980s, Catholic and other voluntary hospitals were bearing the brunt of caring for the uninsured population. In 1983, for example, a study found that urban public and teaching hospitals provided little more than one-third of uncompensated care, while private, voluntary hospitals delivered 60 percent. One approach to health care reform at this time was to increase reimbursements for the poor. To this end, the CHA and AHA favored expanding Medicaid to cover more of the poor population, and both organizations outlined specific changes to Aid to Families with Dependent Children, Social

Security, and Medicaid enrollment rules. In the late 1980s, some Medicaid expansion did occur, mainly restoring cuts made by the Reagan administration in the early 1980s. While this change reduced hospitals' expenditures for caring for the poor, it did not decrease overall hospital costs.[64]

Other Catholic efforts ensued to expand coverage for the poor. When the U.S. Conference of Catholic Bishops' 1981 pastoral letter called for an adequately funded national health insurance program, it drew on Catholic theological views of the post–Vatican II Church. The bishops emphasized the dignity of each human being and access to health care as a basic human right. And if it was a right, then the government had a greater responsibility to guarantee service. The bishops and the CHA declined to endorse a specific insurance proposal, but in the early 1980s the CHA established a task force that eventually released the report *No Room in the Marketplace: The Health Care of the Poor*, in response to Catholic hospital sponsors' continued concerns over meeting the needs of the poor in a tightening hospital market. The document recommended strategies for the Catholic Church and the government to address the needs of the poor, including universal health insurance mandated by the federal government. Another task force developed *A Time to Be Old, A Time to Flourish: The Special Needs of the Elderly-at-Risk*, which advocated policies for long-term care that included integrated health care services and a continuum of care.[65]

One of the dramatic transformations in the Catholic Church after Vatican II was the way Catholics thought about illness: in their 1981 letter, the bishops stated that social conditions such as poverty could lead to physical illness.[66] As noted earlier, prior to Vatican II, Catholics viewed human illness more fatalistically, often viewing it as God's will and as providing stricken individuals with opportunities for grace and redemption. While some of these ideas persisted, the newer view reflected Vatican II's increased emphasis on social justice and human intervention at the societal level.

The Problem of Tax Exemption, Again

Over the last quarter of the twentieth century, as not-for-profit hospitals increasingly became sellers of services yet continued to maintain their tax-exempt status, tensions grew between them and the IRS.[67] From 1956 to 1969, charitable hospitals were required to provide care to the poor. Beginning in 1969, however, the IRS applied the community benefit standard: charitable hospitals had to show that they delivered adequate care to those in their communities who needed their services. It was not required that their main concern be the care of indigent patients, as differentiated from the care of paying patients, but that the entire community receive some benefit from the hospital's operations.[68] In the 1980s, however, skepticism increased over hospitals' values and privileges. In 1986, the Utah Supreme Court ruled that a county tax commission could deny tax-exempt status to a not-for-profit hospital because the hospital did not satisfy the test that it provided free care to the poor equal to its tax-exemption value. The threat to tax-exempt status grew acrimonious as an undercurrent of resentment by hospital leaders surfaced.[69]

In 1989 and 1990, new legislation in the U.S. House of Representatives targeted the hospital industry. If hospitals did not devote a certain portion of their revenues to indigent care, they would face fines and revocation of their tax-exempt status. Specifically, the proposal would impose a $150 billion bond limit for hospitals if indigent care averaged less than 10 percent of total patient care over three years. Emily Friedman argues that some of this was the government's wrapping of its need for money "in the cloak of promoting charitable intent." Yet the government had legitimate financial problems, as needs for schools, education, and other areas grew; it could use the millions of tax dollars not-for-profit hospitals were not paying. Friedman asserts, however, that some government agencies were not suffering for money but just did not believe hospitals were meeting their commitment to the community. Another underlying issue was hospitals' narrow view that they were private institutions, even though most of their income came from public support. Finally, according to Friedman, hospitals believed they were inherently moral because they provided unique moral services, when, in reality, their services were "neither unique nor ethically superior" to other social services. All these issues fed the government's desire to tax not-for-profit hospitals.[70]

Hospitals across the country opposed the legislation, stating that individual institutions and their communities, not the federal government, should decide how to benefit the community. Studies refuted the government's claim that hospitals were becoming less charitable. One showed that voluntary hospitals' uncovered indigent care costs tripled between 1981 and 1989, the same period that not-for-profit hospitals allegedly were becoming more corporate.[71] In 1990 a reporter interviewed Brother Philip Kennedy, president of Alexian Brothers Medical Center in Chicago, who agreed that hospitals should care for those who could not afford it but thought they should not be singled out without requiring all other tax-exempt institutions to provide some kind of free service.[72]

In 1989, the chairperson of the CHA board of trustees, Sister Bernice Coreil, DC, argued against the proposed bill before a House Ways and Means subcommittee. Sister Bernice had a bachelor's degree in business administration and a master's degree in health care administration. She informed the committee that the bill would endanger the financial status of many voluntary, not-for-profit hospitals and thus reduce the availability of care to the poor. When asked what percentage of charity care would be acceptable to her, she responded: "It's not the percent, it's the principle. Where the needs are we will go, and we don't put a percentage on it."[73]

In arguing against imposing a national indigent care criterion on hospitals, Sister Bernice asserted that because Medicaid populations varied from one state to another, providing 10 percent was not possible in some parts of the country. A single national test for charity would not capture the full range of community services a hospital offered. As an example, she cited Seton Medical Center in Austin, Texas. Seton had nearly tripled its charity and community services, from $2 million in 1983 to more than $6 million in 1991, although what percentage of total hospital income these figures represented is unknown. Seton not only provided charity care to more than 7,000 people, but also performed communitywide screenings, held clinics for the poor, donated food each month worth hundreds of dollars, and subsidized health promotion and prevention programs that affected 100,000 people. Yet Seton would not pass the 10 percent test because it had only a 3 percent Medicaid population. This census was affected by the Texas Medicaid system, which covered only persons with incomes of 25 percent or less of the federal poverty level. Thus in Texas, Medicaid was a poor measure of charitable care. Sister Bernice concluded by drawing on logic used by the CHA over the past fifty years: society, government, and churches should share responsibility for funding health care to people in need.[74]

To answer the attacks on not-for-profit hospitals, Catholic institutions became more conscious of the need to accurately reflect their contribution to local communities. In 1988, Catholic Charities of Chicago studied the financial contributions of Catholic institutions in Cook and Lake Counties. For 1986–1987, charity care contributions from the twenty-two hospitals in the diocese totaled more than $203 million as part of yearly operating costs. These included reported and unreported charity care, bad debts, and state underpayments for Medicaid and other welfare patients.[75] In 1989 the CHA created the Social Accountability Budget to facilitate planning for reporting community service. In the preface, it called on the states to face their responsibilities to the people. At the same time, Catholic health care leaders were to raise questions about why charity care was needed in the first place and what role social, political, and economic structures played in causing that need.[76]

The 1990s Environment

By 1992, the country had entered into a major discussion about whether and how to reform the health care system to deal with growing problems of inadequate access and increasing costs. Michael V. Angrosino asserts that Vatican encyclicals on social justice, noted earlier, "were repackaged for the specific context of the U.S. health care reform debate." Indeed, the clergy and laity had been "primed for decades" by papal teachings that "set the moral and philosophical groundwork for health care reform." These encyclicals were written in the context of the longstanding Roman Catholic emphasis on containing the capitalistic market and preventing the exploitation of labor. In addition, respect for human dignity implied respect for the poor and universal access. For their position to be truly Catholic, however, hospital leaders included opposition to abortion as part of the official rhetoric. But other issues were involved. With its huge financial stake in health care through its many institutions, the Catholic Church had a sizeable interest in universal coverage because Catholic hospitals treated large numbers of the poor and uninsured. Cost shifting—the passing of unreimbursed expenses by health providers to private payers in the form of increased insurance premiums—was no longer sustainable. Furthermore, if Congress passed a reform plan that clashed with the Church's ethical values, Catholic hospitals would likely face a severe financial crisis. The CHA, clergy, sisters, and brothers took the position that, even though the debate over the status of abortion as health care was problematic, reform should still be sought.[77]

In 1992, Chicago's Joseph Cardinal Bernardin, a board member of the CHA, called on bishops at the national bishops' meeting in Washington, D.C., to take a greater role in the health care ministry. He acknowledged the problems that might result; as historically bishops' roles in health care had been ambiguous. A few dioceses owned hospitals, but the majority were sponsored by religious communities of women. Debates over the role of women in the Church led some sisters to perceive bishops' interest as interference. To Bernardin, the major challenge was the decline in the number of men and women who owned and administered hospitals, which raised the question of who would continue sponsorship. Second, the structure of multi-institutional systems distanced hospitals from the local bishops. A third challenge was the cutbacks in public funding and the cost-containment strategies of both public and private health care purchasers. Within that fiscal environment, Catholic hospitals were less able to provide care to the poor and uninsured. The last challenge was the growing number of uninsured, which had reached forty million; eleven million were children.[78]

Sister Bernice agreed on the need for collaboration when she addressed the same group of bishops: "Without you there won't be a Catholic health care ministry in the twenty-first century." She noted that in 1984, the major superiors of congregations sponsoring health care had begun a dialogue to address concerns affecting their ministry. Because of the unprecedented challenges to the future of Catholic health care, they expanded that conversation to the whole Church—the hierarchy, religious, and laity. Their collective ability to strategize and set national directions on issues central to the Church's hospital mission was vital. She encouraged the bishops and other hospital leaders to "keep the needs of the poor before the public and try to transform the system of access and financing in favor of the needy and most vulnerable in society." Indeed, women religious and bishops "can be separate no longer."[79]

To that end, sisters and clergy worked with the CHA as key proponents of universal health care access. A CHA Leadership Task Force on National Health Policy Reform headed by Sister Bernice, formed in 1990, set forth a plan entitled "Setting Relationships Right: A Proposal for Systemic Healthcare Reform."[80] It called for integrated delivery networks (IDNs) to link several types of providers in a community so that a broad range of services would be available. The IDNs would offer benefit packages to all persons. State health organizations would distribute a risk-adjusted capitated payment for each individual. A national health board independent of the executive and legislative branches of government would administer the system, whose financing would come from payroll taxes, funds already devoted to state and federal health benefit programs, and other revenues.[81]

The CHA task force aimed to create a vision for health care delivery that would make the CHA a leader in a redesigned, just, and equitable health care system. The CHA board accepted the report, and Sister Bernice presented the plan to the archbishops of the United States.[82] In 1993, the U.S. Conference of Catholic Bishops approved a health care reform resolution that emphasized Catholic values and priorities. Importantly, it was based not on an economic argument but on a moral perspective deemed vital to the political debate: rather than a commodity, health care was a basic right. The bishops offered "a potential constituency of conscience in the midst of a debate too often dominated by special interests and partisan needs." Using the principle of stewardship, the plan demanded attention to duplication and waste that contributed to rising health care costs. Four criteria were basic to any reform plan: priority for the care of the poor, respect for human life from conception to natural death, pluralism in the health care system, and the restraint of health care costs.[83] These principles were in accord with most of President Bill Clinton's health care plan, with one exception: the CHA opposed the inclusion of abortion in the benefit package.

When Clinton was elected president in 1992, problems of the uninsured had become national issues. Hillary Rodham Clinton chaired the President's Task Force on Health Care Reform in 1993, and both she and the president favored managed competition that balanced the marketplace and government intervention. Most important, they supported universal coverage.[84] In January 1993, Sister Bernice, who by that time was senior vice president, System Integration, for the Daughters of Charity National Health System in St. Louis; John Curley, president and CEO of the CHA; and others from the CHA's Washington, D.C., office briefed President Clinton's transition team on the CHA reform plan. Bishop John Ricard of the U.S. Catholic Conference also wrote to Hillary Clinton.[85]

On March 29, 1993, Sister Bernice spoke to the President's Task Force on Health Care Reform. She emphasized the CHA's three pillars of reform: access, quality, and cost containment. Using the rhetoric of exceptionalism, she described the proposal as "uniquely American," a public/private partnership that enhanced the U.S. health care system's strengths while also addressing its weaknesses. Using extensive managed competition, the plan called for combined unitary financing and multiple payers within a pluralistic delivery system, she noted. It was based on explicit values of health care rights, care to the poor, respect for human life, and cost restraints.[86]

Yet Catholic leaders were pursuing a paradoxical lobbying strategy. They urgently wanted universal coverage, but they could not live with a provision for guaranteed payment for abortion and reproductive services.[87] They were convinced that including such payments in any health care reform plan was a "moral tragedy." The CHA argued its position before the White House, Congress, Donna Shalala, secretary of health and human services, and the national press. On April 29, Sister Bernice, Sister Jane Frances Brady, SC, James Cardinal Hickey, and other representatives presented the CHA's full proposal to Hillary Rodham Clinton, expressing their opposition to abortion. According to Cardinal Hickey's report, Clinton expressed "anguish" over abortion and said she did not know how Congress would resolve the issue. She and the president would likely keep their campaign promise to cover medically necessary abortions, but the plan would contain conscience clauses and provisions for Catholic hospitals that recognized state restrictions on abortions. The final Clinton plan used major elements of the CHA's proposal.[88]

In March 1994, the White House invited a delegation of nine CHA members and two hundred other health care professionals to meet with the president and first lady. Sister Bernice, one of three speakers to address the group on the lawn, spoke to the assembled crowd wearing her traditional religious habit, implicitly reinforcing her religious authority, particularly among Catholic believers. In her introduction, Hillary Clinton acknowledged the CHA's work on reform and called Sister Bernice "a leader in making sure each one of us knows health care reform is not just an issue of politics, but an issue of conscience."[89] In turn, Sister Bernice praised the proposed legislation, which provided every American the security of health insurance. She then noted that when the uninsured get care at all, it usually is in the most costly settings. The resulting high costs were absorbed by employers who would find it increasingly difficult to fund insurance coverage for their workers. Thus while she reiterated the moral argument, she also inserted the economic one.[90]

In a radio address on March 26, President Clinton turned up the pressure to support his plan. It was in trouble, and he used all the clout he could muster—including Sister Bernice. The president characterized the content of her address on the White House lawn as "seldom heard in the nation's capital." He paraphrased her remarks: "Health care is about basic human values, about honoring the intrinsic value of every person."[91] Although many Catholics likely heard this reference to "the intrinsic value of every person" as pro-life doctrine, other listeners undoubtedly placed the words in a broader and more generic context. Thus President Clinton and Sister Bernice could present a united front on universal health care without offending their respective constituencies.

At the same time, the CHA continued its press against abortion coverage. In March 1994, Sister Bernice spoke on National Public Radio's *Morning Edition* in a segment entitled "Organized Religion Raises Moral Issues in Health Care." Whereas the Christian Coalition was against the president's plan because of its inclusion of payments for abortion, Sister Bernice thought it was not worth the time and effort to fight over that one issue when so many more important issues were at stake. She believed that any plan with abortion in the benefits package would not get through Congress, because even those who approved of the procedure would not think that people who opposed it should have to pay for it.[92] Catholic leaders in dioceses all across the country used telephone calls, fliers, postcards, and personal visits to Congress to make their two-pronged argument that it was possible to have coverage for all without abortion benefits.The U.S. Catholic Conference, the bishops' public policy arm, distributed fliers to people at church masses advocating this view.[93]

In September 1994, Sister Bernice and several other members of the CHA met privately with Bill and Hillary Clinton. Among other topics, they voiced their concern about the future status of not-for-profit health care and their unease over the commercialization of the hospital marketplace. Hillary Clinton assured the group that the administration would look to CHA for recommendations to protect the not-for-profit hospitals.[94] By then, however, some Catholic parishioners were objecting to universal coverage on the grounds that they should not be obligated to pay for every treatment for every person. To them, it was a huge leap from teaching about human dignity and rights to advocating political positions on universal access. They voiced approval of the obligation to provide access to basic care, but not to comprehensive services.[95] In addition, conservatives and the health insurance industry strongly opposed the Clinton health plan, and Democrats put forth several competing plans rather than uniting behind the president's original proposal. By September 1994, Senate Majority Leader George Mitchell declared the Clinton plan dead.[96]

Cardinal Bernardin evaluated health care policy in 1996, calling it inconsistent and contradictory. Recent health commissions had talked about "a societal obligation to provide access" to care, but a shift had occurred when "the rights of individuals" were replaced by a "responsibility of an undefined 'society'" with competing interests and demands. Known for his commitment to ecumenical and interfaith dialogue, Bernardin called for a rethinking of health care to focus on basic beliefs about the human person and the responsibility of the state. While the tension between an individual's rights and the obligations of governments was healthy, it demanded "rigorous reflection, respectful dialogue, and consensus development."[97] Bernardin died, however, before any further consensus could be built.

In 1997, the Balanced Budget Act reduced payments to Medicare beneficiaries, including hospitals, prompting the CHA to embark on what proved an unsuccessful effort to reverse the changes. Leaders conveyed the message to Congress that the act dramatically limited hospitals' ability to provide care and harmed both patients and hospitals. The U.S. Conference of Catholic Bishops also stepped in, urging Catholics to contact their senators and representatives to restore the cut funds to Medicare. Roger Cardinal Mahoney from Los Angeles wrote the Senate Finance Committee expressing his concerns over the survival of safety-net institutions such as Catholic-sponsored hospitals in rural areas and inner cities. He asserted that Medicare had indeed protected human dignity by assuring health coverage to the elderly and disabled.[98]

For the Church to be most influential in policy, hospital leaders had to demonstrate not only adaptation to the secular hospital market but also support of the Church's tradition of social justice. Thus at the end of the twentieth century, Catholic leaders used the language of rights, access, and advocacy for the poor to define the ideal health care system. This gave them a powerful moral platform and was an example of the Catholic Church assuming the role of moral guardian in U.S. society.

Conclusion

While Catholics often moved cautiously in confronting social prejudices and discrimination, their collective voice for their hospitals received increasing attention and credence as the twentieth century progressed. The public policy arena, a primarily masculine domain but one that Catholic sisters such as Sister John Gabriel Ryan and Sister Bernice Coreil were able to penetrate, opened up a space for Catholic ideals. Catholic hospital leaders constantly updated their hospitals' image as private charities independent of the government as they reasserted their heritage of service and compassion. At the same time, they used the Catholic Church's organizational power and moral authority to influence social policy that affected their hospitals. Sister John Gabriel spoke publicly for the nursing profession and found a voice for herself in this area. She believed that without financial stability, hospitals would not survive, yet survival protection was costly to nurses and other hospital workers whose low wages would continue. Sister Bernice also had a voice in health policy and, despite her conservative position on abortion rights, was quoted by President Clinton, who framed her as a champion of human values.

In the 1990s, Cardinal Bernardin noted that it was imperative that Catholic health leaders measure reform proposals through the lens of stewardship and responsibility. Historically, however, Catholic hospital leaders had actively pursued health policy issues that protected their own concerns, whether it was tax-exempt status, competition with the government, or national health legislation. That Catholic hospitals ideologically preferred to keep the government at bay did not diminish their participation in government programs when it helped their own hospitals to grow.

The bishops' 1993 health care reform resolution stated that the Catholic Church's extensive stake in health care meant that any reform measure should incorporate both public and private hospitals, including religious ones. That line of argument was not new. Throughout the twentieth century, Catholic and non-Catholic hospital leaders tried to head off strong federal policies and regulations by arguing for the value of voluntary efforts. In 1993, the bishops and the CHA expanded the debate by insisting on the values of respect for human dignity and universal access to health care.[99] They continued their advocacy after the Balanced Budget Act passed in 1997. Throughout the debates, the CHA had the organizational structure and power to actively lobby for policies to improve access to care and payment for health care services.

Chapter 6

Harassed by Strikes or Threats of Strikes

"It seems that Oakland would not be Oakland were we not harassed by strikes or threats of strikes," wrote the chronicler of Providence Hospital in Oakland, California, in 1979.[1] Although Catholics were increasingly influential in social justice policies, workplace issues were more problematic. Secular principles dealing with labor applied to service institutions such as Catholic hospitals with religious missions, and over the last quarter of twentieth century, Catholic hospitals became targets for their anti-union stance. Criticism came from within and outside the Catholic Church as strikes occurred in California, Washington, and Alaska. Nurses, other workers, clergy, and sisters as owners and administrators of hospitals were pitted against each other. A number of Catholic hospitals faced up to the labor problem constructively, but unionization in some turned acrimonious.

Many Catholic and non-Catholic hospitals resisted unionization of their workers, mainly due to concerns over the financial viability of their institutions and their objection to having a third party injected into the chain of command. Strong unions significantly influenced hospitals' budgets, which limited management's ability to streamline resources and decrease staffing.[2] When Pope John Paul II visited the United States in 1979, a writer for the *Washington Post* asked: "Will he wonder aloud why Catholic hospitals have reputations for being anti-labor and anti-union?"[3] By the 1990s, debates about workplace justice triggered a reevaluation of the Catholic hospital.

It has been only since the 1960s and 1970s that unions have paid serious attention to not-for-profit institutions such as hospitals.[4] Unions concentrated

in the industrial Northeast, Michigan, and California, with some activity in
Washington and Oregon. It is impossible to say how Catholic sister administrators as a whole felt about unions, because many were in states with restrictive labor laws and never had to deal with them. In other hospitals such as
Seton in Austin, run by the Daughters of Charity, unions were unsuccessful
in 1975.[5] However, unions had a significant presence in the Sisters of Providence hospitals in the West and Northwest.

What made Catholic hospital labor disputes different from others was
that papal encyclicals traditionally supported labor unions. During the late
nineteenth and early twentieth centuries, when U.S. Catholics were in the
bricks-and-mortar period of building hospitals, churches, and schools, the
labor movement was organizing industrial workers. The Catholic Church's
pro-labor attitude resulted from management's reluctance to recognize the
basic rights of workers, many of whom were immigrant Catholics, until workers formed their own associations. Pope Leo XIII's 1891 *Rerum Novarum* (Of
New Things) recognized unionization as a social right, emphasizing the
duties of both workers and employers: workers were to respect property and
avoid violence, and employers were to provide a just wage, safe working conditions, and reasonable working hours. In 1931 Pope Pius XI's *Quadragesimo
Anno* (After Forty Years) developed Pope Leo's teachings further. Issued in
the middle of the Great Depression during the rise of communism, it condemned both socialism and communism for their materialism and totali-
tarianism and also attacked the unfettered competition of capitalism that
burdened the working class.[6] Pope John XXIII in 1961 issued *Mater et Magis-
tra* (Mother and Teacher) about Christianity and social progress, which supported a just wage but implored workers to use collective bargaining rather
than strikes. The 1965 Vatican II document *Gaudium et Spes* (Joy and Hope)
taught the value of human labor and maintained that workers had the right
to join unions. Then in 1981 Pope John Paul II issued *Laborem Exercens* (On
Human Work), which stated that workers had a right "to form associations
for the purpose of defending the vital interests of those employed in the various professions."[7] In 1991, on the hundredth anniversary of *Rerum Norarum*,
he issued *Centesimus Annus* (Hundredth Year), which proclaimed the cultural importance of unions.[8]

"The Privilege of Service": 1930s–1950s

In the early and mid-twentieth century, both public and religiously based
hospitals spent an enormous amount of time consolidating their power over

their employees.[9] They took advantage of their nursing students, who usually lived in hospital housing and were exploited as a labor force. Most hospitals, including Catholic institutions, did not hire the nurses they graduated until around 1940. Rather, graduate nurses worked either in public health or in private duty in homes or hospitals. Students and graduate nurses all experienced poor working conditions, toiling six to seven days at a time, working twelve hours a day, and in the case of students, receiving little or no pay.[10]

Some nurses unionized in the early twentieth century, but during the 1930s unions grew in number across a variety of job sectors, enhanced by the National Labor Relations Act (Wagner Act) of 1935 that legally sanctioned organization for the purpose of collective bargaining. Voluntary not-for-profit hospitals, including Catholic facilities, paid employees less than prevailing rates and tried to keep unions out of hospitals. As Rosemary Stevens notes, hospital leaders asserted that their facilities played a special role in serving the community, "that their low pay was a virtue, since it attracted staff who were motivated by the 'right values.'" Nurses and other workers put patient care above their desire for better wages and cherished the "privilege of service," hospital leaders claimed, extending the traditional dedicated service of Catholic sisters to all hospital workers. These claims kept wages low and unionization out of hospitals until well after World War II.[11]

Although only a small number of nurses joined unions, they influenced the American Nurses Association (ANA) leadership in 1937 to form a Union for Nurses Committee. Ultimately, however, the ANA rejected trade unionism; its leaders asserted that nursing was a special service role for women rather than one that sought self-interest or money.[12] Opposition to unions also existed among rank-and-file nurses, fed by nativist and class prejudices. For example, a nurse from Seattle claimed: "If one wants to be ruled by an alien who is practically illiterate, join a union and discover what real bondage means."[13]

After World War II, the severe nursing shortage that had developed during the war did not abate. Registered nurses' salaries lagged far behind those of other workers, and many nurses believed that their low salaries and poor working conditions contributed to a poor quality of nursing care. While the ANA vacillated, some graduate nurses elected not to wait for their national leaders and began joining labor unions.[14] In Seattle in 1946, Local 126, the Nurses and Professional Workers' Union of the American Federation of Labor (AFL), helped nurses negotiate with the Seattle Hospital Council for a minimum salary of two hundred dollars per month and a forty-hour workweek. Nurses at Saint Luke's Hospital in Seattle even won the right to have a closed union shop (nonunion members had to join within a specified period of time after being hired).[15]

Nurse leaders eventually took advantage of union pressures and hospitals' dislike of unions: in 1946, the ANA House of Delegates initiated the Economic Security Program (ESP), which endorsed collective bargaining to improve nurses' employment conditions. It also maintained that the state nurses' associations should be the sole representatives for nurses in areas of labor relations.[16] Nurses in the western states were among the leaders in negotiating contracts to further their rights as workers. Indeed, a precedent had been set in California in 1943 when the California State Nurses Association began representing its membership through collective bargaining in negotiations with employers.[17]

Yet nurses' longstanding commitment to public service and national health needs strongly influenced the ANA's ESP policy. It did not demand changes in social, economic, or gender relations, and it did not operate as a typical labor union that stressed fair labor practices and a living wage. Instead, it emphasized professionalism and strengthening the health care delivery system. Following this philosophy, nurses agreed not to strike under any circumstances. Thus the policy distanced professional registered nurses from tactics used by other unionized workers.[18] The ANA and its state organizations viewed themselves as professional associations, and they represented only registered nurses. On the other hand, Local 1199, the National Union of Hospital and Health Care Employees, represented pharmacists, technicians, therapists, and maintenance workers. It was established in 1932 and in 1998 would affiliate with the Service Employees International Union.[19] The line between professional organizations and unions was blurred, however; some registered nurses and physicians eventually joined other unions.

In 1947, in response to rising union radicalism, Congress enacted the Labor-Management Relations Act, or Taft-Hartley Act, which restricted the activities and power of labor unions; it banned closed shops, campaign contributions, and other union practices. Taft-Hartley exempted not-for-profit hospitals from coverage under the act, however, because of their quasi-public role, which meant they did not have to bargain collectively with their workers. Despite this exemption, some state nursing associations such as Washington's and California's were strong enough to represent nurses effectively.[20]

Labor Policies in Catholic Hospitals

In 1935, after the National Labor Relations Act legally sanctioned collective bargaining, Sister John Gabriel Ryan, SP, of the Sisters of Providence in Seattle discussed attitudes toward labor unions with other hospital leaders. Their opinion was overwhelmingly in favor of pursuing a neutral policy. They agreed that hospital wages, hours, and working conditions in their own and other hospitals were deplorable, and that bettering wages and living conditions would be a strategic move to prevent the formation of unions.[21] They also predicted, accurately, that personnel problems would be dominant subjects for hospital administrators over the next several years.[22]

Throughout the 1940s, the Catholic Hospital Association (CHA) consistently resolved that Catholic institutions should take the lead in fostering reasonable and just working conditions and salaries for all employees.[23] Dialogue over workplace issues continued in the next decade. In 1950, Father John Flanagan, executive director of the CHA, acknowledged that Catholic hospitals sometimes did not remunerate workers sufficiently. He also spoke to the issue of job security, asserting that qualified people were often arbitrarily dismissed when a religious sister or brother became available for the their position. Promotion was limited for those who were not members of the religious congregation, because the important positions such as supervisors were filled by the sisters and brothers, even if they were not qualified in experience or education. He also noted that laypeople in Catholic hospitals were capable of making institutional policies and that having them do so would increase their loyalty to the organization. This participation did not mean that they would assume too much control.[24] Leaders in Catholic hospitals were slow to follow Flanagan's advice.

Understandings of the Church's role in labor and health care changed in the 1960s with Vatican II's increased emphasis on justice and human dignity, which coincided with rising health care expenditures. Conflicts and alliances followed between Catholic and secular hospital workers and leaders as the federal government, the Catholic hierarchy, and unions increasingly became involved in hospital decisions. Labor activist Monsignor George C. Higgins, former director of the Social Action Department of the U.S. Catholic Conference, criticized Catholic hospitals' anti-union activity. Hospital managers countered that unions interfered with their ministry to local communities.[25] Since relatively few Catholic hospitals were affiliated with dioceses, they were not under the control of local bishops. Rather, the majority were independently owned by religious orders of women who did not always agree with the bishops.

Labor Strikes in Washington and California

In the 1940s, Providence Hospital in Seattle saw frequent time-consuming negotiations between administration and nurses over labor contracts. These negotiations involved the Washington State Nurses Association (WSNA), an organization with an aggressive government relations program since 1909 when it first lobbied the state legislature to pass a Nurse Practice Act. In 1938, the WSNA adopted a resolution that discouraged any affiliation with trade unions, but within two years general-duty staff nurses were expressing dissatisfaction over low salaries and poor working conditions. Although many nurses viewed the ANA's Economic Security Program and collective bargaining as inappropriate for professional nursing, in 1948 the WSNA officially adopted its own Economic Security Program and recommended that it be the sole collective bargaining agent for its members.[26]

As early as 1950, union activity showed up at Providence Hospital in Oakland, California, along with the other hospitals in the Bay Area. Providence managed to avoid serious problems until 1958, when members of Local 250 of the Hospital Workers Union of nonprofessional workers walked off the job for twenty-one days. Reports of employees being jostled and threatened appeared in the newspaper and in the sisters' hospital chronicles. Although a wage agreement was reached and the hospital reemployed the strikers, the union did not win its demand for a closed union shop. The Sisters of Providence valued the loyalty of their workers who did not strike, and the settlement made them more careful in their screening of applicants.[27]

In the 1960s and 1970s, inspired by the women's movement, nursing unions increased in the western states. A critical situation occurred in San Francisco in 1966: two thousand dissatisfied nurses resigned from several hospitals during a dispute over their labor contracts. To subvert the ANA's no-strike policy, the San Francisco nurses resigned en masse.[28] Soon after resolution of the problem, the California Nurses Association (CNA) broke with tradition and the ANA by endorsing strikes as a means of obtaining economic goals.[29]

Providence Hospital leaders averted similar problems with registered nurses in 1966 by agreeing to a fact-finding panel on wages and salaries that consisted of national Catholic and lay arbitrators of labor management disputes. But management and nurses deadlocked in 1969 after many months of trying to negotiate a new contract with the CNA. A two-week walkout resulted; in June, ninety registered nurses left their jobs. The administrators of the Associated Hospitals of San Francisco and the East Bay, of which Providence was a member, offered a raise in salaries. The main issues, however, were the CNA requests for patient care committees, an outside arbitrator if agreement could not be reached in disputes, and increased vacation time.[30]

Hospitals already had broadly constituted patient care committees that included doctors, administrators, nurses, and other specialized personnel. But these members were appointed by the administration, and CNA demanded that they be elected by CNA staff nurses and that disagreements be submitted to an outside third party for fact finding. "No hospital—or any other properly-managed organization—can agree to such a method," the hospital lawyer claimed. "This . . . infringes upon the function of governing Boards of Trustees who have the final authority, responsibility, and accountability (moral, financial and legal) for patient care."[31]

As the strike persisted into its second week, the mayor of San Francisco intervened and called in a state mediator. On July 2, 1969, Sister Francis Ignatius, SP, administrator of Providence Hospital, wrote her superior: "Yes, thank God, the strike is OVER! As expected in negotiations, each side has to GIVE something. However, the strikers are to be called back only as our census grows and the numbers warrant coverage." The negotiating sessions had gone into the early hours of the morning. "I'm still *convalescing*!?!?" she wrote.[32] In addition to salary raises, the nurses won increased vacation time and the right to elect staff nurses to the patient care committees of each hospital belonging to the Associated Hospitals of San Francisco. In another compromise, disagreements would be referred to a group consisting of the CNA director or her representative, a staff nurse, and two members of hospital management.[33] Hospitals were not necessarily hurt by strikes or threats of strikes; their strategy was to renegotiate with insurance companies to increase their reimbursements to pay for higher room rates for patients. They threatened to cancel contracts during negotiations with insurers, but often they ended up making deals before the contracts expired.

In the 1960s, reverberations over the labor struggles among nurses in California occurred up and down the West Coast. Some AFL-CIO union representatives, labeled "agitators" by the sisters, stationed themselves at the exits of Providence Hospital in Seattle, urging the nurses and other workers to join a union. Compounding the situation, over the course of the spring and early summer, many of the hospital's nurses and other workers left to work at Boeing Aircraft Company, where they could get higher wages. To the Sisters of Providence, it was a case of "big business" luring away their workers, because "money talks."[34] The irony was that money certainly talked for the sisters as well, with one significant difference. Whereas the secular nurses understandably focused on money that went into their paychecks, the sisters' money concerns related more to hospital operations and budgetary balance sheets. They were not responsible for earning an income to pay rent or feed children, but they were keenly aware of income needed to purchase supplies and pay creditors.

To stave off union leaders looking for new fields to organize, Seattle hospitals, including Providence, agreed to give registered nurses an increase in salary before they asked for it.[35] In 1967, however, more than 1,200 of the 1,700 registered nurses in the twenty-two Seattle-area hospitals signed conditional mass resignations in protest of the Seattle Hospital Council's proposed labor contract. Nurses still lagged behind teachers and secretaries in pay and benefits. In response to the nurses' demands, Providence Hospital administrators met with representatives of the WSNA. Averting the threatened resignations, management agreed to a nursing pay increase of one hundred dollars a month, health and welfare benefits, workers' compensation, and Social Security.[36] Ninety-five percent of all Providence employees received wage increases that averaged 10 percent, which increased hospital costs by $550,000 the first year, increased charges to patients, and led to renegotiations with insurance companies to pay higher patient costs.[37]

The 1970s and 1980s

Hospital leadership was especially tested in the 1970s as nurses' strikes increased, even though nursing incomes had slightly improved over the previous decade. In 1969, for example, Bureau of Labor statistics reported that the national average salary of a full-time general-duty nurse was $141 for a forty-hour week, compared to $129.51 for most production workers, although lower than schoolteacher salaries.[38] Furthermore, government-imposed wage controls and hyperinflation in the 1970s eroded incomes for nurses and many others.

In June 1974, 4,400 members of the CNA went on strike in forty-three Bay Area hospitals, including Providence Hospital in Oakland. The nurses promised to cover emergency, intensive care, and coronary care units, but most of the operating room nurses and one-third of Providence's general-duty nurses walked out. The hospital cancelled all elective surgery and operated at only half capacity.[39] According to the Providence chronicler: "The nurses wish to control the staffing patterns with the hospitals which cannot legitimately be given them as responsibility for patient care rests fundamentally with the administration."[40] According to the nurses, however, the issue was having greater input in controlling patient care. To one nurse, administrators could not deal with "relinquishing any kind of input to the nurse."[41] Nurses particularly sought changes in how hospitals used their skill and knowledge, and they wanted to end the practice of placing unskilled nurses in intensive and coronary care units.[42] The ANA, holding its convention in San Francisco at the time, pledged its support for the strike. But one editorial questioned how picketers could be serious about having patient interests at heart when they were really telling patients, "The nursing attention you're not getting today is really for your own good."[43]

Caspar Weinberger, U.S. secretary of health, education, and welfare, intervened and a federal mediator stepped in. On June 25, 1974, after twenty-one days off the job, CNA members voted to end the strike. In addition to salary increases and improved health benefits, the new contract reaffirmed the nurses' previously held rights to participate in staffing decisions but reiterated management's prerogatives and rights in the area of staffing. Nurses won another round when management agreed that nurses without appropriate specialized training would not be used in critical care areas except for training purposes and emergencies. Both the California and the American Hospital Associations drafted statements that challenged nurses' demands for control of staffing. To them, only hospital administrators should have the responsibility to determine the number of employees, their qualifications, and their assignments within the institutions.[44]

The San Francisco strike attracted national attention, and only six weeks later Congress amended the Taft-Hartley Act. On July 26, 1974, President Nixon signed the bill that permitted nurses and other workers in not-for-profit hospitals to use collective bargaining and strikes. Union representation elections in hospitals increased, leading many hospital managers to reevaluate their labor-management programs to deter the formation of unions, and hence strikes.[45] At the same time, Catholic Church leaders began taking a deeper look at hospitals' anti-union activities. In 1975 Reverend Kevin O'Rourke, O.P., director of the CHA's Department of Medical-Moral Affairs, wrote "Christian Responsibility for Labor and Management." Because Catholic hospitals were part of the Church's ministry, he stated, they were obligated to apply Church teachings that called for protecting human dignity and seeking unity between labor and management. The importance of Catholic social teaching was that it offered "instructions and guidance concerning social and economic problems . . . [but] seldom will there be only one 'Catholic' solution to a particular problem." After describing the pro-labor history of the Catholic Church, O'Rourke went on: "If unions impede human dignity, or if human dignity can be achieved without unionization, then the value of unionization comes into question. In other words, unionization is a relative rather than an absolute good." He asserted that some pro-labor clergy and social agencies that criticized Catholic hospital management were unaware of the social and economic forces that health care facilities faced.[46]

Union activity gained further attention in Seattle in the 1970s, when the city suffered a severe economic recession, mainly because Boeing, the city's largest industry, had nearly halved its labor force of more than eighty thousand. Providence Hospital became involved in the first nurse's strike in the history of Washington in 1976. The WSNA initiated it against fifteen of eighteen Seattle area hospitals, with more than 1,800 nurses participating in the ten-week strike. Nurses wanted raises in salary, better staffing, and an end to sixteen-hour work shifts on the grounds that better working conditions would ultimately improve patient care.[47]

The strike, which began at 7:00 AM on July 12, 1976, was effective in keeping registered nurses from going to work. The Seattle Area Labor Council sanctioned the strike, and local trade unions promised they would not cross picket lines.[48] Nursing supervisors, head nurses, licensed practical nurses, aides, and other nonstriking nursing personnel covered the units. The hospital reduced admissions to emergency cases only, and elective surgery became very selective. In addition to the nurses, members of Local 900, the Retail Clerks International, also struck the hospital. These included medical technologists, pharmacists, occupational therapists, physical therapists, and dieticians. On July 30, the hospital reluctantly began layoffs and shorter workweeks due to the low patient census.[49]

On August 1, nurses at Group Health Cooperative, a consumer-controlled health care system in the Seattle area, also began a strike, which lasted twenty-eight days. They, too, organized within the WSNA.[50] Fearing that the strikes would spread further, Providence Hospital managers held their ground against the nurses: "We realize that giving in to excessive demands by WSNA for wages and changes in working conditions now will only cause other groups to exert pressures for concessions."[51]

In the negotiations, hospitals relaxed somewhat on salaries but not on other issues. The WSNA called for just cause for termination to be determined by a third-party arbitrator, but Seattle hospitals believed this would eliminate their rights as employers to dismiss someone for incompetence; employees could already take complaints to a hospital grievance committee. The major point of contention, however, was mandatory membership of all registered nurses in the WSNA. The hospitals objected to that closed shop, stating it would burden part-time nurses who could not afford the hundred-dollar annual dues. If nurses refused to join, their employers would have to terminate them. Providence management iterated its support of unions but its opposition to mandatory membership: "We feel it would be morally irresponsible to deny the right of any employee to freely decide to be represented by a union or belong to a union or pay a service fee to a union." Their records showed that 40 percent of the registered nurses in the Seattle hospitals were not members of WSNA. According to the WSNA proposal, if these nurses did not pay the dues, they would be fired. Sisters and other administrators believed that mandatory membership in the WSNA was the real issue for the nurses and that the other complaints were just a smokescreen.[52]

After sixty-eight days, the strike finally ended on September 17, 1976. In a three-year contract, nurses received an 8 to 12 percent pay raise the first year and a 6 percent raise the following two years. Seventy-four percent of the affected nurses ratified the contract. More than eighty of the striking nurses lost their jobs, however, due to a decrease in patient census, although they received first priority for openings as the census increased. Records are silent about the union shop, but it appears that it did not succeed.[53] Throughout the next two decades, Providence management succeeded in warding off strikes. While negotiations with unions sometimes lingered on for months, management set up yearly evaluations to solicit employee input regarding job satisfaction and subcommittees to address the issues, and they insured that nurses were represented on different hospital committees.

In the 1980s, as hospitals diversified their services and Diagnostic Related Groups (DRGs) changed Medicare reimbursements, private hospital employees' average hourly wages increased 23 percent as wages decreased 6 percent for other employees in the private sector. Registered nurses benefited most, receiving the highest wage increases of all hospital workers. Hourly earnings increased by 17 percent between 1981 and 1989. Other highly skilled workers such as therapists and pharmacists also saw growth in earnings, but wages for nonprofessional occupations such as admitting personnel, clerks, cleaners, and food service workers stayed flat across the decade.[54] The proportion of union members in all labor sectors was falling, but nurses in the West and Northwest were becoming more active.[55] Although a serious shortage of registered nurses led hospitals to raise wages, as in the past wages and salaries were not the only concern. The shift to health maintenance organizations had reduced hospital stays everywhere, while hospitalized patients were more seriously ill and required more intense nursing by skilled personnel. Nurses had more work to do in less time, and they criticized hospital corporations for sacrificing patient care to the bottom line. These conditions led more hospital workers to seek union representation.[56]

Other strikes occurred at Sisters of Providence hospitals. After one especially contentious strike in 1986 at Saint Elizabeth's Hospital in Yakima, Washington, one physician opined in a letter to the editor: "Service *professionals* are not primarily concerned with their own 'rights' and personal interests. The traditions of caring for others, which are best exemplified by Saint Francis, Florence Nightingale and Sister Gamelin [founder of the Sisters of Providence] are not upheld by abandoning the sick and denying care to the poor." This physician thought it "foolishness" that nurses who carried signs on picket lines that stated, "Scabs, we will never forget," could see themselves as professionals. If they wanted more money, they should have gone into another field.[57]

Nurses took the physician to task. One commented: "Your salary has been cut by 10 percent and your benefits reduced! What would you do?" She turned to the rhetoric of service, stating that the "patient's health [is] the center of our focus." Another woman took a different stance, reminding readers that Florence Nightingale "made waves" as she advocated for the principles of good nursing care. Who could say what she thought about nurses striking? She likely would have objected to inadequate staffing because it hurt the patients and was unfair for nurses. To this writer, nurses' professionalism "does not mean being meek, subservient and unwilling to speak out, but rather that is a role expected of nurses by others, such as administrators and doctors." If medicine had progressed beyond the horse-and-buggy days and received proper payment for its services, why not nurses? Indeed, nurses deserved financial recognition: "For those who relish thoughts of nursing as being a holy calling, gratifying and glorious in and of itself, expecting the duties to be performed without any concern for finances, I say, how do you take that to the bank and pay bills with ideals and little else?" A third nurse responded that she did it for patients so that she could have the education, competence, and time to give them the best possible care; for her family, so that she could assure them a decent honest wage; and for future patients, who deserved a registered nurse at the bedside. She concluded: "Yes, I was a nurse on the picket line. And Florence Nightingale was probably by my side."[58]

In 1987, three hundred registered nurses walked out of Providence Hospital, Oakland. Throughout the strike, the hospital administrator, Sister Dona Taylor, SP, wrote memorandums to all employees explaining why

Providence could not meet the CNA's demands. She posted financial figures on cafeteria walls to show that the hospital had lost $250,000 in the first quarter of 1987, with losses over the second quarter predicted to be even greater.[59] Nurses countered that it was appropriate for hospitals to cut costs, just not in nursing.[60]

Financial problems at Providence in Oakland and competition with Merritt Peralta Medical Center in the city led to their merger in 1992, creating Summit Medical Center. While the Sisters of Providence no longer owned the hospital, their representatives still served on the Summit board of trustees. The CNA backed a costly forty-five-day strike that year, and the formidable labor movement in the East Bay Area and its allies in government took the strike public. Presidential hopeful Jerry Brown proclaimed solidarity with the strikers, and Jesse Jackson helped arbitrate.[61] Nurses appealed to the Sisters of Providence corporate headquarters in Seattle for support, but the nuns opted not to get involved with management. Summit received scathing publicity from the newspapers and a state congressional hearing over its refusal to go to arbitration, its attempts to break the unions, and its failure to ensure adequate care to patients during the strike.[62]

"Nurses Will Not Strike Based on Money": The 1990s

Hospital restructuring affected nurses' workloads and control over their work. During the 1990s, as hospital leaders underwent tough negotiations with managed care providers to keep costs in line with revenues, registered nurses accounted for much of the labor cost. In 1996 and 1997, they represented approximately 23 percent of the hospital workforce.[63] To lower operating costs, hospitals frequently replaced registered nurses with unlicensed personnel.[64] Although wages had increased in the 1980s to attract and retain nurses, one survey showed that by 1994, 27 percent of hospitals that were cutting back on costs did so with nurses as the target. Other studies showed that lower staffing levels did, indeed, lead to more positive financial performance, and policy makers hailed this achievement.[65]

While hospital finances improved, nurses' working conditions suffered. The nurses at Providence Hospital in Anchorage, Alaska, voted to unionize with the Alaska Nurses Association in 1994 after Providence executives launched a reorganization effort to reduce expenses by $10 million over the next two years; nurses feared for their jobs and worried about drastic changes in working conditions.[66] Nearly five years later, the nurses still did not have a contract. They struck the hospital on April 15, 1999, with the Alaska Nurses

Association as their bargaining unit. Nurses were caring for far more patients than they thought safe and particularly wanted more input into staffing in areas that affected nurse/patient ratios. Management continued to claim that it was the administrators' right to make staffing decisions.[67]

The program director for the Alaska Nurses Association stated that "nurses will not strike based on money" but for better patient care. Prior to the strike, the *Anchorage Daily News* on April 4 had reported on a study of nine hundred hospitals that showed Providence nurses with higher salaries than three out of four hospitals in the country. But many of the nurses' salaries had been frozen since they voted to unionize in 1994. Union members believed Providence earned plenty of profits, enough to compensate the nurses with higher salaries.[68]

Yet throughout the strike, nurses centered their attention on patient care issues. As health professionals, they were genuinely concerned that there simply were not enough nurses to meet increased work demands.[69] And their strategy worked. After two weeks, a federal mediator stepped in, and talks began anew on May 6 and 7, 1999. This time, nurses received exceptional community support, including that of Teamsters Local 959, the International Association for Firefighters Local 1264, and physicians. It was also at this time that Linda Aiken, Eileen Lake, Julie Sochalski, and other researchers were providing evidence of significant links between nursing education, nurse staffing, patient deaths, and preventable complications.[70]

On May 10, after twenty-six days of the strike and five years of labor discord, nurses and management reached an agreement that nurses overwhelmingly supported. While they received only slightly higher pay, they won the right to have pay increases based on years of experience. They also obtained more say in patient care, limits on mandatory overtime, and the right to be notified at least three weeks before the hospital made major staffing changes involving nurse/patient ratios; the notice would then go to a committee consisting of four nurses and four hospital representatives. Nurses wanted medical benefits after retirement, but they did not get them.[71]

Catholic Healthcare West

Established in 1986, Catholic Healthcare West (CHW), based in San Francisco, operated hospitals in California, Arizona, and Nevada. In the 1990s, CHW became involved in especially contentious debates with unions. The company's roots date to 1857 with the founding of Saint Mary's Hospital in San Francisco by Mother Baptist Russell of the Sisters of Mercy (now of

Burlingame). Mother Baptist, an immigrant from Ireland, and her sisters took charge of the county hospital during a cholera epidemic. They quickly learned the value of payment for hospital services when the county did not pay them what they needed to care for 140 patients. Mother Baptist told the county supervisors to assume responsibility for payment or she would open her own hospital. She did so in 1857.[72]

Catholic Healthcare West was unique in its collaboration of several orders of Catholic sisters, who formed the system to pool resources and increase their buying power for supplies and services. As part of its corporate system, CHW also acquired many secular hospitals. It was representative of the large not-for-profit hospital systems, being the eighth largest in the nation and the largest not-for-profit hospital chain in California.[73]

CHW partnered with hospitals and physicians, and in July 1996 it placed under single management Saint Mary's Medical Center and Saint Francis Memorial Hospital in San Francisco, Seton Medical Center in Daly City, and Seton Medical Center Coastside in Moss Beach. The four hospitals and their doctor-group affiliates had 655 active physicians, 4,100 employees, and annual revenues of $334.6 million. Together, they admitted 27,500 patients in 1995, which was 17 percent of the market share in San Francisco and surrounding counties.[74] Professional lay hospital managers were responsible for daily administration. While Catholic hospitals advertised their missions as delivering quality and compassionate care, in 1996 leaders of the state's health care unions accused CHW managers of undermining community service in order to build their empire. The West Bay CHW's new CEO countered: "We're in a competitive business, and like any competitive business we need to address productivity." For the fiscal year ending in June 1996, CHW reported a net profit of $160 million and a Standard and Poor's bond rating of A+.[75]

Shortly after that year's annual report was published, on August 13, 1996, 370 health care workers of Service Employees International Union (SEIU) Local 250, consisting of licensed vocational nurses, dietary workers, clerks, housekeepers, and technicians, staged a one-day strike at Saint Mary's Medical Center and Saint Francis Memorial Hospital to protest stalled contract negotiations. The union asserted that the merger of the four CHW hospitals in July hurt workers economically and impaired patient care. The CHW board had just announced $2 million in budget cuts and the subcontracting out of linen and laundry departments at the two hospitals. The union also demanded that, because the hospitals made huge profits, their not-for-profit status be revoked. According to the *San Francisco Examiner*, the CHW president received more than $1,550,000 in salary and benefits for the two fiscal years ending in June 1995. Between 1992 and 1994, his compensation had increased 58 percent.[76]

The executive director of the California Nurses Association also went to battle with CHW. "The nonprofit vs. for-profit distinction is a farce by and large," she told the *San Francisco Chronicle*. "They all use the same [anti-union] consultants." In April 1997, CHW settled a two-year contract with the CNA. At two Catholic hospitals, Saint Mary's in San Francisco and Daly City's Seton Medical Center, the agreement gave nearly five hundred nurses a 4 percent raise over two years, maintained existing benefits, and introduced domestic partners coverage. Nurses at two other Catholic facilities received raises to bring them into parity with Saint Mary's.[77]

Unionization efforts spread to Sacramento in 1996 as SEIU Local 250 attempted to organize licensed practical nurses, some registered nurses, house-keepers, and other workers at seven CHW hospitals. The SEIU went public in accusing CHW of harassment and intimidation of pro-union employees with help from an anti-union consulting firm. The union's president said he preferred dealing with the for-profit Columbia/HCA over CHW. "They're really no different in their business philosophy, in the way they provide care or the way they treat workers," he said, but at least the Columbia chain admitted to being driven by the bottom line.[78] The issue sparked a national debate among Catholic sisters, brothers, and clergy about the Church's role in labor disputes. In 1998, a religious brother and spiritual director at one of the Sacramento Catholic facilities asked: "Is it a mortal sin to believe that unions are not the best way of social justice? Employees have a right to unionize, but they clearly have a right not to unionize." Other Catholic clergy accused CHW management of hiring a consulting firm that had a reputation for union busting. Management denied any charges of intimidation, arguing that the hospital hired the management firm to help employees decide whether to unionize or not.[79]

In June 1998, nurses at Mercy Healthcare Sacramento, an affiliate of CHW, participated in a one-day strike to protest what they characterized as low salaries and a shortage of nurses. The spokesperson for Mercy said the CNA was asking for a 28 percent increase in salary over three years, much more than the hospital could afford, since it had lost $8.5 million the previous year. While hospital leaders asserted the workers' right to choose unionization or not, they believed it was not in the workers' best interest. Rather, the "most constructive relationship between management and non-management employees is a direct one."[80] Mercy Healthcare of Sacramento eventually settled with the nurses, but CHW then demanded higher reimbursements from Blue Cross. They reached a last-minute agreement in July 1998; and although the details were not publicized, one can assume that they involved increased hospital reimbursements.[81]

In 1998, CHW expanded into the Los Angeles area, the most competitive health care market in the country, by acquiring eight non-Catholic facilities. By then, the federal Balanced Budget Act of 1997 had cut payments to hospitals. Leaders at CHW found themselves owning overpriced physician properties and hospitals that often overlapped in services.[82] Consequently, CHW suffered severe losses from overexpansion. The hospital system ended the 1999 fiscal year with a $353 million loss and a significant reduction in its bond rating, from A+ to BBB+.[83]

Other alliances occurred between labor and the Catholic Church in Los Angeles, where in September 1999 pro-labor themes dominated church services. Whereas the white European portion of the Catholic Church had prospered, the Latino population was less well off. Especially targeted for unionization were many Latinos who were blue-collar workers in Catholic hospitals. At the oldest Roman Catholic Church in the city, the pro-labor priest yielded the pulpit to a union organizer, who in Spanish asked the large Latino crowd for its support of unions at three Catholic-owned hospitals. These included Saint Francis, Saint Vincent's, and Robert F. Kennedy Medical Center, which, according to the organizer, had not responded positively to unionizing efforts. Another church with a large diverse population prayed for workers who were exploited by large corporations pursuing cheap labor. The hospitals pointed out, however, that 30 percent of their workforce already belonged to unions. Los Angeles's Roger Cardinal Mahony issued a statement asking both sides to agree to arbitration by a neutral third party, but his plea was unsuccessful.[84] The SEIU invited clergy to meet with workers at Saint Francis Hospital, but, according to one source, when they arrived they were escorted by hospital security to the meeting place, where hospital supervisors quickly surrounded them; consequently, few workers were willing to speak. A few weeks later an Episcopal priest was barred from entering the hospital with a delegation. According to the same source, efforts to reach out to the sisters involved in management failed.[85]

Unionization in California hospitals had mixed results. After a long battle, hospital employees at five Sacramento CHW hospitals voted against the union in January 2000. In February, the SEIU won the right to represent three hundred licensed vocational nurses and respiratory specialists at

Saint Francis and Robert F. Kennedy in Los Angeles; but other workers there in March 2000 voted against joining the SEIU. An SEIU spokesperson said employees were intimidated; but a spokesperson for CHW asserted: "This vote showed the workers believed in the hospital and wanted to continue the direct relationship."[86]

Three months later, the CHA held its annual meeting in San Francisco; the SEIU picketed the association. Protesters distributed copies of a videotape that accused CHW of ignoring Church teachings on labor rights. Estimates of the number of protestors varied from two hundred to six hundred. One journal article asserted that the SEIU tried to "annoy, embarrass and hector the hospital system into recognizing new labor units in Northern and Southern California," criticizing the union for ignoring an agreement to tone down tactics. By then, CHW had severed its relationship with two anti-labor consulting firms. A spokesperson for Mercy Healthcare Sacramento expressed her frustration: "It's perplexing to us how SEIU's continuing efforts to undermine our mission and service to the Sacramento community could possibly benefit the community or our employees."[87]

On July 6, 2000, the largest ever one-day hospital walkout occurred in San Francisco when four thousand SEIU members protested worsening patient care conditions in CHW and Sutter Health facilities. Hospitals then in the CHW system included Saint Mary's Medical Center and Saint Francis Memorial Hospital in San Francisco, Seton Medical Center in Daly City, and Summit Medical Center Oakland, which had recently merged with the Catholic Providence Hospital in that city. The strike came as 1,730 nurses were in the fourth week of a walkout at two Stanford hospitals. According to one newspaper, more than 60 percent of hospitals in California, where managed care had made great inroads, were operating in the red.[88] Both sides took their issues to the public on the air and in print. A worker at Saint Mary's complained that her employer was oriented to the bottom line rather than to patients. Another asserted that hospital corporations took over community hospitals and cut staffing and services, all the while taking millions of patient care dollars out of the community to fuel their corporate expansions.[89]

By then, CHW was restructuring, having survived significant financial losses as the government cut reimbursements, the number of uninsured increased, and health insurers lowered reimbursement rates. Blue Cross blamed the losses on the company's rapid expansion.[90] Union officials noted that CHW could afford to pay its CEO $800,000 a year while its workers were the lowest paid in the Bay Area. A spokesperson for the health care industry commented that unions never understood that their real enemy was the purchaser of health care, not the hospitals, but she agreed that there were legitimate workload issues.[91]

Both sides claimed victory after the one-day July walkout. Members of the SEIU were pleased that so many workers had united against the hospital corporations, whereas the hospitals were satisfied that they had stayed open and maintained their emergency rooms. Yet many of the striking workers could not return to work immediately, because the hospitals had hired temporary replacements and cut down significantly on patient admissions. Consequently the strike cost workers significant income, while the hospitals had to pay millions of dollars to replacement workers.[92] Less than a month later, on August 3, 2000, SEIU employees walked out again on CHW and other hospitals. The strikes were becoming so numerous that public health officials feared a state of emergency as the winter months neared and more people got sick. A trend was developing in which, as one official claimed, "what otherwise is a routine labor dispute turns into a potential public health care crisis."[93] The one-day strike ended without resolution, and over the next several months, other walkouts occurred, culminating in a statewide strike in December when eight thousand SEIU workers in twenty-two hospitals walked off their jobs to protest employers giving them no voice in patient care.[94]

"A Fair and Just Workplace"

Battles between the union and CHW created headlines all along the West Coast between 1996 and 2002. One Catholic publication noted that the confrontations placed Catholic sisters, most of whom had ceded control over their hospitals' day-to-day operations to lay managers, in a "no-win situation." In July 1999, three thousand Catholic activists in Los Angeles met at the Catholic Gathering for Jubilee Justice and publicly supported the union. Monsignor Higgins breakfasted with AFL-CIO president John J. Sweeney. Higgins, long known for his labor activism, thought that one reason sisters and Catholic hospital administrators were reluctant to confer with pro-union priests and bishops on the issue of unionization was their longstanding discontent with the male domination of a patriarchal Church.[95] He also criticized the sisters' hiring of anti-union management consultants, which he could not reconcile with Catholic social teachings. Specifically, he listed the U.S. bishops' 1986 pastoral letter, "Economic Justice for All," that supported employees' rights to organize and bargain collectively, which had stated: "Basic justice demands that people be assured a minimum level of participation in the economy. It is wrong for a person or a group to be excluded unfairly or to be unable to participate or contribute to the economy. . . . Work with adequate pay for all who seek it is the primary means of achieving basic justice in our society."[96]

Leaders at CHW countered criticism by noting that they defended their workers' rights to choose. But management not only had to see that care was provided but also had to balance budgets, meet payrolls, be good stewards to their resources, and maintain facilities. In addition, in exchange for their tax-exempt status, not-for-profit hospitals were expected to provide charitable services to the poor and uninsured. For example, sisters at CHW ran a community grants and loan program that funded local nonprofit organizations dealing with low-income housing and job training.[97]

Disputes over unions eventually led to a reevaluation of Catholic hospital policy. In 1999, Sister Mary Roch Rocklage, RSM, nurse and CEO of Mercy Health System in St. Louis, initiated work on a new document. On August 26 of that year, under Sister Mary Roch's guidance, a subcommittee of the U.S. Bishops' Domestic Policy Committee released "A Fair and Just Workplace: Principles and Practices for Catholic Health Care." It summarized a two-year dialogue between major superiors of Catholic congregations, other Catholic health care leaders, bishops, and organized labor. The document acknowledged the tensions that framed the major issues in Catholic health care, which involved the religious mission of Catholic hospitals and their need to operate in a market-oriented economy shaped by public policy and available resources. "Catholic health care is not just another economic activity or project; it is a demonstration of our faith and a commitment to human life and human dignity," it stated. In an effort to find common ground between workers and health care leaders, it called on management to structure the workplace and steward limited resources so that employees could have what they needed to carry out their work. It also supported workers' right to freely choose to participate in a union or not, and suggested that if workers chose unionization, management should negotiate in good faith. All parties should "promote a collaborative workplace of participation, harmony, and mutual respect for the roles of workers and management as well as to advance the provision of health care as a fundamental good." Workers, too, had a responsibility for ensuring that the mission of Catholic health care was not compromised, whatever choices they made.[98]

The Domestic Policy Committee released the document as a working paper rather than as a formal statement. As such, it did not mandate action but offered ideas for dialogue, reflection, and action. The CHA welcomed the statement: "Too often attention is focused on local labor disputes without equal attention to the countless communities where Catholic health facilities and workers, whether unionized or not, relate well," it announced. The CHA acknowledged the pain and frustration that all Catholic health care leaders experienced as they tried to be faithful to the ideals of Catholic social teachings as fiscal resources diminished. Catholic hospitals were charting new territory as they navigated organizing efforts, and it was especially disheartening for them to be alienated by other members of the Church.[99]

"A Fair and Just Workplace" found limited consensus, with some religious superiors questioning why only health care was targeted and not other services such as schools. Others believed it assigned greater obligations to Catholic hospitals than to unions.[100] The value of the document, however, lay in its challenge to study and put in place whatever was needed for a just work environment, and to continue the dialogue. It provided guidance for hospital boards, sponsors, administrators, employees, and labor union leaders on how to find ways to be more open and less confrontational.[101]

Around the same time, the National Interfaith Committee for Worker Justice published a booklet of guidelines to help hospitals and unions move toward dialogue. The Catholic sisters and ecumenical leaders with extensive experience in health care administration who developed the booklet acknowledged management's concern over how to honor compensation and staffing arrangements when they proved too costly, given government and insurance reimbursement rates. Some hospital leaders feared that unions would destroy faith-based health care. Others found negotiations with union representatives a time-consuming process and thought grievances could be handled through existing hospital structures. The guidelines challenged both unions and management to engage in good-faith dialogue rather than adversarial relationships. After the booklet's publication, some religious hospital leaders thought the document favored unions too much, while others thought it did not go far enough for workers.[102]

Yet results were under way. After several years of contentious negotiations, strikes, and public charges and countercharges on radio and in newspapers, in April 2001 Catholic Healthcare West and the SEIU signed an agreement on procedures and conduct for union elections that covered forty-five CHW institutions in California and Nevada. Called "historic" by Monsignor Higgins, it promised to pursue joint efforts to influence health care policy in several areas: universal access to affordable health care, greater rights for immigrant workers, and more federal and state health care coverage for children.[103] The following year the SEIU reached a contract agreement with CHW that covered nine thousand workers in the California and Nevada hospitals. A CHW spokesperson reported: "I think we decided it's probably in our best interests to work with SEIU. We signed a similar agreement with the California Nurses Association in February. We felt this was something that would benefit both of us if we went about it the right way."[104]

Overall wage and benefits increased, and all regular workers received medical insurance that the employer fully paid. The agreement also made CHW the first major hospital system in the West to offer dependent health care coverage to families, spouses, and partners of all full-time employees. To address the high turnover and shortages of nurses and other staff, the agreement established joint union-management committees to work out staffing issues. "It means I have a voice," said one registered nurse who sometimes had to care for as many as fourteen patients at a time.[105] The new agreement also allowed employees the right to organize without interference from the hospitals. The major bones of contention throughout the battle had been short staffing and workload problems. Under the new terms, any dispute over staffing would go to an outside arbitrator, a complete turnaround from the last several years.[106]

In 2002, Sister Patricia Talone, RSM, PhD, was vice president for Mission Services with the CHA. She had earlier served as ethicist for the Mercy Health System in Philadelphia and as vice president for Mission Services and ethicist for Unity Health, a subsidiary of the Sisters of Mercy Health System in St. Louis.[107] In "Labor and Catholic Health Care," published in 2002, Sister Patricia traced the historical context in which the Church's stance toward labor developed, reminding her readers that nineteenth- and early twentieth-century Church teachings on labor focused mainly on industrial workers, not on those in the service sector, making their application to health care a challenge. "After all," she wrote, "a Catholic health care organization does not merely deliver a product; it commits itself to a ministry," with the primary goal not to make money but to care for the poor, sick, and vulnerable, although financial strength was needed to carry out this mission. She explained how Catholic hospitals were a community of people dedicated to working together toward a common goal, unlike the usual dichotomy of employer-employee. Thus when arguments got contentious between management and employees, people inside and outside the ministry became discouraged.[108]

Sister Patricia took the history of the Church's social teachings a step further, noting that as early as the 1830s Catholic leaders in Europe had encouraged workers' associations. In the United States, however, Catholic clergy initially forbade membership in the Knights of Labor, a large union formed in the 1870s, because of its being a secret society and their fear that membership would weaken Catholic workers' allegiance to the Church. Church leaders also were concerned that the violence and intimidation from other unions in the nineteenth century would lead to anarchy.[109]

Acknowledging that the papal encyclicals supported unions, Sister Patricia described a broadening of the Church's concern over labor and social justice in the mid-twentieth century. First, in 1967, Pope Paul VI in *Populorum Progressio* (On the Development of Peoples) declared that unions were acceptable as long as they were committed to workers rather than to materialism or atheism. Pope Paul eschewed the exclusive pursuit of material possessions, while at the same time insisting that employees be involved in dialogue to build a community of workers. Then, in *Octogesima Adveniens* (A Call to Action), he argued in 1971 that labor solutions were multifaceted and should be approached on a regional basis so that the involved persons could determine what was best for each area. Furthermore, as Sister Patricia quotes the pope: "In concrete situations, and taking account of solidarity in each person's life, one must recognize a legitimate variety of possible options. The same Christian faith can lead to different commitments." In his 1991 *Centesimus Annus* (Hundredth Year), Pope John Paul II supported unions but also expressed concern over growing consumerism. He followed his predecessors in urging both workers and employers to be responsible in creating dialogue and harmony.[110]

Sister Patricia zeroed in on the sisters' major concern: while Church teachings continued to have relevance, "whole communities rise or fall, depending on whether their Catholic health care institutions survive and flourish." Disharmony in these institutions could lead to alienation not only of administrators and workers but also of patients and local residents. Most important, this would endanger the entire ministry. Her historical review of the Church's social teachings revealed that they were never static. And while the encyclicals issued calls for dialogue, they also included warnings that unions might demand too much. Workers had the right to join or not to join unions. "But workers, unions, and management alike must recognize that greed, violence, intimidation, and coercion are totally unacceptable because these actions tear down rather than build up the community." Furthermore, "it would be presumptuous to suggest explicit applications for health care trustees and administrators."[111]

Sister Mary Roch, who had initiated discussions on "A Fair and Just Workplace," chaired the board of trustees of the American Hospital Association as well as the board of the Sisters of Mercy Health System. In 2003, she admitted that "maybe in some areas we [sisters] passed the baton too quickly. I think there may be some remedial work to do. . . . When we took on the mindset of corporate America, we began to talk that way, we looked that way, we acted that way and we alienated our own selves and our employees. We were acting like 'we are market-driven,' versus, 'we are in the market but it doesn't apply to us.'" While Catholic hospitals had an eye on the bond market where they gained their financing, they needed to pay more attention to the Catholic mission of providing good care, especially to the needy. "We may need to talk the corporate language on the street [Wall Street], but among ourselves we have a different language. . . . We are about stewarding and ministry."[112]

After nearly ten years of dialogue, leaders from Catholic health care, the labor movement, and the U.S. Conference of Catholic Bishops agreed in 2009 on another set of principles to facilitate fair practices when health care workers decided whether or not to join a union. According to *Respecting the Just Rights of Workers: Guidance and Options for Catholic Health Care and Unions*, issued by the bishops, it was up to workers rather than hospital managers, bishops, or union leaders to decide whether or not to unionize.[113]

In the midst of these negotiations were Catholic sisters sitting on boards of directors of local hospitals who often found themselves at odds with other board members on these issues, especially when it came to executive salaries. When sisters left hospital administration and became active at the board or trustee level, their governance duties focused more on strategies than on operations. As board members, they had a say in hiring CEOs and vice presidents, and they helped set executive salaries under the guidance of a human resources consultant. While objective market data dictated what the salaries would be, Sister Helene Lentz, CSJ, found setting salaries one of the hardest things to do as a board member of several of her congregation's hospitals. To her, executive compensation in health care was too high, considering the low salaries of others such as dietary and housekeeping workers: "I understand the need to pay executives in a manner consistent with their counterparts in other health care institutions, so I always went along with the recommendations . . . but it deeply troubled my conscience." When she expressed her concerns to the board, she often felt powerless, since "other board members and executives tend to think sisters don't really live in the 'real' world so don't understand the financial matters of a family," which Sister Helene admitted might be an "accurate perception." When it came to other matters of Church relations, however, sisters were much more influential. Lay board members often let nuns take over in matters relating to mission, values, and ethics.[114]

Conclusion

The tangled involvement of hospitals and unions in the last half of the twentieth century revealed tensions over hospitals' religious missions and the business realities within which they operated. As nuns' numbers declined and lay administrators grew in power and influence, some Catholic labor supporters thought the sisters were unduly deferential to these laypersons. While the sisters' national leaders operated in an oversight capacity toward the administrators, they were reluctant to exercise their authority in local administrative matters. Nuns as board members could express concerns about issues just as any other board member could, although they often felt they had no influence. Unions were also vying for power at this time, since there was fierce competition among different unions to expand their membership.

All these factors undoubtedly resulted in many of the sisters struggling with inner conflicts between their religious ideals of social justice and inclusiveness and their personal desires for independence in decision making. Although they embraced principles of fair treatment for hospital workers, it was often difficult to trust that such treatment could be administered without their guiding hands. And because they were imbued with their sense of mission and considered themselves on the side of the poor and vulnerable, it was difficult for them to accept criticism from their workers.

Debates about workplace justice helped trigger a reevaluation of the Catholic hospital. The dispute involved clergy and labor leaders, who criticized the sisters for what they believed was a conflict between the Church's traditional social teachings and the way the nuns dealt with unions in their hospitals. In particular, clergy who did not have to administer or sponsor hospitals differed with sisters who did over how to interpret the teachings. Sister Patricia Talone and other sisters argued for a more nuanced understanding that Catholic hospitals existed as part of their local communities. Collaboration among workers and employers was necessary to build up the community. Sisters understood their work not only as socially useful but also as part of a religious obligation. They asserted that the Church's teachings never attempted to provide definitive answers for each situation but offered moral guidance for decision makers.

Physicians and hospital managers had criticized the nurses over the years for striking instead of cultivating the feminine value of self-sacrifice. Even though nurses negotiated privately for higher salaries and better benefits, they determined that their best public strategy was in fact to underplay these personal demands; because they believed patient care had been dangerously compromised, they emphasized instead the needs of their patients, particularly safety issues stemming from inadequate staffing and the need for more and better hospital services. While in the 1970s and early 1980s, studies had not yet shown conclusively that actual harm to patients came from increased nursing workloads, nurses believed that they did. As workloads became less manageable, nurses wanted a greater voice in patient care. To increase the legitimacy of their claims, they framed their argument as a concern over their patients rather than over their own salaries.

Such strategies might have suggested that nurses were acquiescing, playing traditional feminine roles that frowned on self-serving motives and open confrontation, but this was not the case. Rather, their labor negotiations were based on strategic decisions designed to maximize their chances of success. There is ample historical evidence of nurses' willingness to confront authority and self-advocate. But they turned the strong messages they were hearing from doctors and the public sentiment that stressed nurses' sacrificial service over material gains to their advantage. In essence, they found the approaches that offered the best results, forgoing the moral battles that would yield little more than pious satisfaction.

Nurses did not have accurate data on workload issues until researchers such as Aiken and her associates showed, first, that adequate nurse staffing did indeed prevent patient complications and deaths and, second, that nursing burnout and job satisfaction were related. At last, evidence supported nurses' longtime concern about these issues.

When Catholic Healthcare West reported a $307 million loss after 2000, it restructured and divested itself of almost all of its physician practices and some of its hospitals. The more financially sound Daughters of Charity hospitals had been among the strongest in the system; collectively they had broken even in 1999. To increase their inside decision making and have more control over the health care of the local communities they served, the Daughters pulled out of their affiliation with CHW in 2001 and took back management of four hospitals in the Bay Area and three in Los Angeles.[115] They formed their own system in 2002, with most of the operating functions residing in the individual hospitals. As part of the large CHW system, their money had been pooled, yet as one Daughter of Charity stated: "The money we have is the money of the poor; it isn't our money." The Daughters also wanted to be able to care for anyone whether they had insurance or not rather than committing funds to financially strapped hospitals.[116]

Meanwhile, CHW renegotiated contracts with insurers such as Blue Cross for higher reimbursements. It diversified into ambulatory care areas and markets with bright prospects for growth, such as Phoenix and Las Vegas, locating its largest investments in areas that provided only a modest charitable service relative to the entire CHW chain of hospitals. With its mission perspective, CHW also decided to stay in areas such as Los Angeles where the social needs were greatest, renovating or replacing facilities that offered the most charitable services, although it did not expand into areas with high economic and health-related needs. Operations at CHW improved, resulting in gains of $183 million in 2005 and an A- bond rating. Most of the hospitals now are unionized and the workplace has stabilized.[117] In their 2002 agreement, CHW made decisions that substantially improved their relationships with unions. Importantly, they expanded health care coverage to many new groups, thereby enhancing their commitment to universal access to health care.

Chapter 7

Practical Solutions to Complicated Problems

On February 4, 1999, the *Wall Street Journal* noted growing tenion between religious and medical practices. Its front page, quoted Reverend Gerard Magill, priest, ethicist, professor at St. Louis University, and paid consultant on policy development to the Daughters of Charity and other religious sponsors of Catholic hospitals: "This may shock you, but the Catholic Church is very keen on finding practical solutions to complicated problems. We certainly will not do immoral acts, but we can certainly come to arrangements."[1] Catholic hospitals would not allow abortions, but other services such as those dealing with reproductive technology might be open to further discussion. In the last decades of the twentieth century, as ethical issues developed over the growth of biotechnology, and many Catholic hospitals were partnering with non-Catholic facilities, tensions developed that challenged Catholic identity. To counter these threats, bishops and the Vatican became more influential in hospital decisions.

According to Magill, abortion and assisted suicide were "nonnegotiable" issues in Catholic hospitals, but certain ethical precepts could guide religious leaders as they discussed reproductive services. To Magill, the key to whether or not services such as sterilization could be performed was physical distance; that is, a controversial procedure could be provided if it was done at a site not owned or financed by a Catholic facility. Quoted in the same *Wall Street Journal* article, Sister Bernice Coreil, DC, executive assistant to the president of the Daughters of Charity, took the same tack: "People see the church as one-dimensional and rigid. There is no cookie cutter which says, in this situation, this is what you do."[2]

That Catholic hospitals should be flexible in order to continue their health care mission was one side of the story. Another view came from Catholic critics who held that any association with secular partners that allowed reproductive services to continue undermined Church teachings. Thus Magill's statements did not go uncontested. One Catholic physician responded that "'fine distinctions' simply erase an institution's Catholic identity and Christian witness before the public. . . . If the significant pressures of the marketplace make the sisters feel like a gun is to their head, sometimes the answer must be: 'Go ahead and shoot—I cannot deny my God or my faith.'" Another writer opined that while abortion and assisted suicide were nonnegotiable and "black and white," perhaps "much else is gray, but need it be dirty gray?"[3] Such critics included the Vatican, which altered or halted several hospital mergers and partnerships. Yet a third position was held by supporters of contraception and abortion, who worried that women's rights were being usurped.[4]

The National Context

Market forces continued to transform the financing and delivery of health care in the 1990s, as we have seen. In 1996 alone, a record number of hospital affiliations occurred, involving 768 hospitals compared to 650 hospitals in 1994, many of them Catholic providers. Table 7.1 shows 131 affiliations of Catholic hospitals between 1990 and 1996 according to type of ownership of the partner. As noted, close to 80 percent involved affiliations with secular, non-Catholic partners—66 percent with non-Catholic, not-for-profit hospitals or systems and 12 percent with for-profit groups.[5]

Reproductive technologies such as sterilization and in vitro fertilization were emerging as particular areas of conflict, since the Catholic Church forbade such procedures. The language itself was objectionable to John M. Haas of the National Catholic Bioethics Center: "Lower animals reproduce; human beings procreate," and the entire phrase "reduces everything, even the most intimate of human relations, to the level of manufacture, mass production, and economics in a technological and capitalist society."[6] These tensions created a dilemma that affected not only Catholics but also non-Catholics, physicians, nurses, and their patients—and the majority of physicians, employees, and patients in most Catholic hospitals were not Catholic.

Table 7.1 **Catholic Health Care Provider Affiliations, 1990–1996**

| | Ownership of Affiliating Facility | | | |
Year	Catholic	Non-Catholic not-for-profit	Non-Catholic for-profit	Total
1990	1	1	0	2
1991	2	2	1	5
1992	1	4	0	5
1993	1	1	0	2
1994	3	18	6	27
1995	8	31	7	46
1996	13	29	2	44
Total	29 (22%)	86 (66%)	16 (12%)	131 (100%)

Source: "Is There a Common Ground: Affiliations between Catholic and Non-Catholic Health Care Providers and the Availability of Reproductive Health Services?" #1322. The Henry J. Kaiser Family Foundation, November 1997. Used with permission. http://www.kff.org/womenshealth/1332-catholic3.cfm. Accessed December 1, 2009.

The Vatican Context

When a Catholic facility sought affiliation with a non-Catholic institution, it had to seek approval from the local bishop, who was not usually involved in hospital policy decisions in the independently owned and operated Catholic hospitals. As a cleric and bishop however, it was his responsibility to communicate directly with the Vatican's Congregation for the Doctrine of the Faith, which was responsible for ensuring that Catholic teachings were implemented in all Church facilities.

It is important that this story be understood in the broader context of national health care issues. While the Catholic Church historically hailed the positive accomplishments of scientific medicine, leaders tempered their appreciation with concern over potential religious and moral consequences. What is now called bioethics arose out of an ancient practice of medicine among whose major tenets was commitment to the welfare of the patient.[7] Not until the eighteenth century did Christian theologians, including Catholics, begin to develop a body of literature on the topic. In the late nineteenth and early twentieth century, topics such as eugenics, euthanasia, abortion, and reproductive sterilization drew the most attention. In the nineteenth century, Catholic moral theology began to forbid abortion during all phases of pregnancy, although the Church allowed therapeutic abortion to save the life of the mother until the latter half of the nineteenth century.[8] In his 1930 encyclical *Casti Connubi* (On Christian Marriage), Pope Pius XI explicitly forbade abortion, and bishops at Vatican II and Pope Paul VI also condemned it. Since then, exceptions have been approved for pregnant women with uterine cancer and ectopic pregnancies, for example. Although Catholic hospitals could not perform abortions, they did not actively oppose its performance in other hospitals.[9]

The first written set of medical ethical norms for Catholic hospitals came in 1920 from the Archdiocese of Detroit; it dealt with surgical procedures and prohibited anything that resulted in sterilization or the destruction of fetal life. Many other dioceses accepted this one-page code and hung it on the operating-room walls of their hospitals.[10] In 1947, Catholic leaders published a revised *Code of Medical Ethics for Catholic Hospitals* and two years later, the *Ethical and Religious Directives for Catholic Health Facilities* (hereafter cited as *Ethical and Religious Directives*). Each was revised again in the 1950s.[11]

The politics of abortion and birth control were related. While Catholic lobbying did not influence an 1873 law banning the distribution of contraceptive devices through the mail, Catholics became active from the 1920s to the 1960s in opposing the loosening of restrictions on access to birth control in the United States. For example, Catholic leaders helped defeat legislation in the 1920s that would have permitted public advertisements of birth control products, and over the next two decades they opposed laws permitting the opening of birth control clinics. They also helped limit physicians' authority to prescribe birth control. Pope Pius XII in 1949 rejected artificial insemination of women as immoral.[12]

In the 1950s, as biomedical techniques gained ground, Catholic theology that linked religion and health care as a ministry underpinned the views of many bioethicists, and Catholic theologians took a leadership role in debates in this arena. Yet as society increasingly secularized, there was a shift away from this religious center.[13] In the 1960s birth control became a central debate topic among U.S. Catholics, and a rapidly increasing number of clergy and laity began to doubt traditional Church teachings on the issue.[14] The debate heated up in 1968 when Pope Paul VI's encyclical *Humanae Vitae* (Of Human Life) reiterated the Catholic Church's stance against birth control, which caused a serious divide between the Church and laity and split the Catholic clergy.[15] Studies showed that only a fourth of the laity agreed with the Church's stance on sexual reproductive issues.[16]

Furthermore, debate over the proper use of biotechnology in the 1960s fragmented U.S. society, especially over questions about human life. Among the debated bioethical issues were those concerning technically assisted reproduction and abortion. As all sources of authority, including religion, were called into question in the 1960s, tensions grew between the religious origins of bioethics and what bioethicist Edmund D. Pellegrino calls an "anti-religious trajectory of modern culture." As a significant number of Catholics and members of other religious faiths felt less allegiance to their church teachings in the 1960s, they also were "dazzled by the promised utopia of biotechnology," Pellegrino suggests. When bioethical issues became matters of public policy, the Catholic Church felt it imperative to step in and address points that were in conflict with Catholic beliefs.[17]

Following Vatican II, bishops became more active in the fray. The National Conference of Catholic Bishops (NCCB) focused on internal ecclesiastical concerns regarding Church policy. Composed of all members of the Roman Catholic hierarchy, its work included rulings on the issues of abortion and reproductive services in Catholic hospitals. In 1971, the NCCB came out with a new version of *Ethical and Religious Directives*, which carried additional weight in light of the 1973 Supreme Court decision in *Roe v. Wade* that legalized abortion. While the document did not settle the issue of whether sterilizations could be performed when necessary to avoid diseases arising from pregnancy, the Vatican barred this very procedure in 1975 in *Quaecumque Sterilizatio* (Responses on Sterilization). In 1986, Chicago's Joseph Cardinal Bernardin promulgated a "consistent ethic of life" that expanded the debate over abortion to include the sanctity of human life in many areas—genetic counseling, capital punishment, modern warfare, and the care of the terminally ill.[18]

Further complicating the situation were disagreements within the Church itself. In 1984, for example, a coalition of U.S. sisters criticized the hierarchy's attempts to make abortion illegal. Criminalizing abortion would not do away with the procedure but "would make safe abortions only available to the rich," they stated. Also that month, ninety-seven Catholic activists, including some nuns, signed a newspaper advertisement in the *New York Times* that supported the right of Catholics to dissent with the Church's ban on abortion. The Vatican threatened the sisters with expulsion from their religious congregations, but their superiors did not dismiss any of them, although two eventually left their congregations.[19] The Church bishops officially responded to new reproductive technologies in 1987 in their "Instruction on Respect for Human Life in its Origin and on the Dignity of Procreation," or *Donum Vitae* (The Gift of Life). This document taught that an intervention was moral if it "assists the marriage act to attain its natural end; if it *replaces* the marriage act, then it is immoral" (emphasis in original).[20] Thus in vitro fertilization was rejected. *Donum Vitae* also labeled as abortion the destruction of pre-embryos, and it aimed to influence not only Catholics but also national legislation on biomedical issues.[21] The *Ethical and Religious Directives* were revised again in 1994. The revision, according to Sister Jean deBlois, CSJ, and Reverend Kevin O'Rourke, OP, suggested, among other findings, that "church teaching on respect for the dignity of the person stands in clear contrast to the prevalent secular notion that people earn or achieve dignity when they pass some arbitrary milestone, physiological or otherwise." As the *Ethical and Religious Directives* emphasized, it was respect for the dignity of the human person that inspired "an abiding concern for the sanctity of human life."[22]

A New Partnership

A series of events involving Seton Medical Center in Austin, Texas, highlights the clash of medical technology, economics, and Catholic moral teaching in the United States in the last quarter of the twentieth century. On May 4, 1995, Charles J. Barnett, president and CEO of Seton, announced an agreement between Seton, a Catholic facility owned and operated by the Daughters of Charity, and the City of Austin, which owned Brackenridge Hospital (see figure 11).

Seton Medical Center was part of the Daughters of Charity National Health System, one of the five top-ranked hospital systems nationally. Good intentions and a desire to preserve Catholic health care were the Daughters' primary motivating factors as they wrestled with whether to allow the public hospital to continue providing reproductive services. Under the agreement, Seton would take full management and control of Brackenridge, a public facility with primary responsibility to care for the medically indigent, which had accumulated $61 million in debt. Losing Brackenridge's services would mean a significant loss to the community. The explicit purpose of the transaction was to "ensure the continuation of essential health care services, including trauma, women's and reproductive services, and children' services, for all citizens of Austin and Travis County, regardless of their financial means."[23]

Seton committed to pay $10 million up front and $2.2 million annually to lease Brackenridge's buildings and consolidate services, which would make Seton the city's largest hospital system.[24] In turn, the city would pay Seton

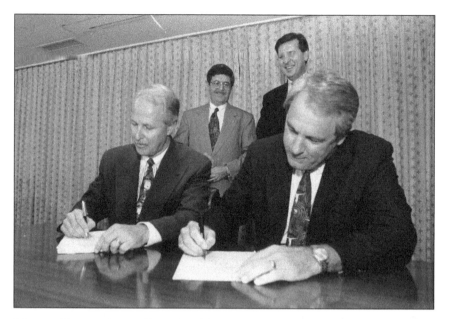

Figure 11   American College of Healthcare Executives fellow Charles J. Barnett, *left*, signs the Brackenridge/Seton agreement, alongside Austin City Council member Ronney Reynolds; *standing*, Austin city manager Jesus Garza, *left*, Bruce Todd, *right*. Austin, Texas, ca. 1995.

Courtesy Seton Family of Hospitals, Archives Division, Austin, Texas.

$5.6 million annually for charity care provided at Brackenridge. This public/private partnership was not unusual, but part of a trend toward overall consolidation in the hospital marketplace. What complicated it was that Seton had to adhere to the *Ethical and Religious Directives* developed by the U.S. Conference of Catholic Bishops (USCCB) in 1994, which banned direct involvement in reproductive services to which the Catholic Church morally objected. Specifically, these services included contraception, sterilization, abortion, and infertility services such as in vitro fertilization and artificial insemination. Yet, the *Ethical and Religious Directives* permitted an indirect role in the delivery of some of these services, should a Catholic hospital affiliate with a non-Catholic institution.[25]

As a condition of the lease, Brackenridge insisted that its reproductive services be maintained, except for abortions, which had all along been referred to an outside provider. Key to this agreement was that Brackenridge retain ownership of its facility, and that Seton not identify Brackenridge as a Catholic institution. Because of this important stipulation, and after consultation with Catholic ethicists and theologians, Seton announced that "in recognition of the community's need for reproductive services, those . . . that are currently available at Brackenridge will be retained."[26]

The compromise between Seton and Brackenridge brought national attention as mergers and affiliations involving Catholic and secular institutions continued. In 1998 alone, the Catholic Health Association (CHA) reported thirty-two such partnerships; other sources put the number as high as forty-three.[27] The partnership between Seton and Brackenridge was a lease arrangement rather than a merger, but the conflict of views and values that ensued involved all the players and characteristics of the national debate—the Vatican's direct involvement, Catholic criticism of the Daughters of Charity, intense deliberation over the provision of emergency contraception, and compromising attempts at solutions.[28]

Abortion—always a divisive issue—again became part of the national dialogue in the 1990s as President Bill Clinton included reproductive care in his health plan.[29] Opponents and a small but powerful Christian Coalition had joined the dispute and inserted family planning in the abortion debate. Particularly disconcerting to supporters of family planning was the growing elimination of reproductive health services when Catholic hospitals merged or partnered with secular institutions, which reduced access to care for individuals needing and wanting those services.[30] Women's religious congregations, whose aims were to meet the needs of the most vulnerable and poor, found themselves in conflict with the Catholic Church's directives proscribing reproductive services. Women's rights activists in Austin joined the Brackenridge discussion and insisted on being part of the decision-making process.

Austin Health Care Context

When the Daughters of Charity established Seton Hospital in 1902, they had a special concern for the sick and poor, which they renewed under the profound influence of Vatican II. An essay by James L. Connor describes the change in sisters' ministry emphasis: they no longer saw themselves as bringing students and patients into the nuns' world but rather as "entering into *their* world, to share *their* experience."[31]

Brackenridge, too, had a commitment of community service to the poor. Established in 1884, it was the oldest public hospital in Texas, and in 1995 it had the only trauma center and the city's only graduate medical education program. As Brackenridge's long-standing financial problems came to a head, its administrator, aware that it could not survive as a stand-alone hospital, asked the Daughters of Charity to submit a proposal: how might Seton assist the city's operation of Brackenridge and of city-owned Children's Hospital of Austin to make them more competitive in the Austin hospital marketplace?[32]

Religious commitment to the poor and market forces in Austin influenced the way the Daughters, lay leaders, and bishop responded. The for-profit Columbia/Hospital Corporation of America (HCA) chain had changed the health care landscape in Austin when it took over four independent, full-service hospitals in the area: Columbia/HCA now owned nearby Round Rock Hospital and South Austin Medical Center; it partnered with the Austin Diagnostic Medical Center that was under construction; and it was solidifying a partnership with Saint David's Medical Center, originally affiliated with the Episcopal Church. In the face of these changes, the Daughters of Charity and the city of Austin as owner of Brackenridge agreed that some form of consolidation was mandatory for the survival of each hospital. It was projected that Seton's payments to Brackenridge over thirty years would allow the city to pay its hospital debts and leave a $38 million balance.[33]

Two national studies raised fears that Columbia/HCA would not treat the medically indigent should Brackenridge close its doors. One reported that eighty-six hospitals in twenty-two states had been cited by the government for refusing to treat emergency indigent patients for nonmedical reasons in 1993 and early 1994.[34] Another study examined the impact of a California public hospital's closing on patients' access to health care: a significant number of uninsured patients were denied access to care elsewhere, and the closing was associated with a decline in their health status.[35] Most important, then, the partnership between Seton and Brackenridge would maintain the safety net for the medically indigent, a goal long embraced by both health care institutions.

Some citizens, however, were concerned that a private hospital's management of Brackenridge would remove it from public scrutiny. One member of Brackenridge's advisory board lamented: "When you can do things behind closed doors—you can decide who gets care and who doesn't—I assume the worst is going to happen." In addition, 520 Brackenridge employees signed a petition opposing the lease. They wanted to remain city employees, and they believed that the city had not sufficiently explored alternative funding. City Manager Jesus Garza admitted that Seton's management of Brackenridge would remove the hospital's public accountability. To solve this problem, the city council appointed a board to oversee Seton's responsibility for the city's indigent health care programs.[36]

Material Cooperation

After the city council approved the lease in May, final acceptance had to come from the Seton board of trustees and its parent organization, the Daughters of Charity National Health System in St. Louis, to whom all Seton's religious and lay administrators and trustees were ultimately responsible. Prior to a final decision and public announcement, however, the Daughters of Charity and Bishop John McCarthy of Austin consulted with four leading medical ethicists and Monsignor William Broussard, executive director of the Texas Conference of Catholic Health Facilities and vicar general for the Austin Diocese, to ensure that the lease arrangement was in compliance with the *Ethical and Religious Directives*.[37] The Daughters in St. Louis questioned Monsignor Broussard about the challenges an agreement between a Catholic and non-Catholic hospital would bring. Noting his consultation with canon and civil lawyers, Broussard replied: "First, they felt that a lease arrangement would not mean ownership in the strict sense;"—ownership would remain with Brackenridge. Second, "a lease arrangement does not give the facility a Catholic identity, but rather gives the lessee certain rights and privileges."[38]

The Austin diocese sponsored public meetings to sell the deal to local Catholics and area clergy. Broussard and Magill prepared a position paper to explain the reasoning behind the Seton/Brackenridge partnership from the perspective of Church teachings and ethical principles. Their argument built upon the Catholic tradition of social justice and the 1994 *Ethical and Religious Directives*, specifically, Directive 69, which stated that Catholic institutions could participate in networking arrangements that included cooperating, in a limited way, with the provision of services such as sterilization that Catholic teaching prohibited, although this did not include abortions.[39] The *Ethical and Religious Directives* justified the principle of "material cooperation," and it was this principle that was used to clarify Seton's position. Material cooperation "permits a person to cooperate in some way in a wrong procedure," ethicist David F. Kelly explains. It does not excuse "wrongdoing" but enables limited cooperation with other parties who engage in wrongful acts "as long as certain conditions are met." Had the Daughters of Charity agreed with the idea of sterilization and in-vitro fertilization as morally "right," and had they intended to be active in the provision of reproductive procedures, then they would be guilty of "formal cooperation." In formal cooperation, which was always wrong, the cooperator desired that the wrong act be performed, according to Kelly. "But all of us are at one time or another caught up in some form of cooperation with actions we consider morally wrong." Catholic tradition says that "material cooperation is morally right . . . if the good effects to be realized . . . outweigh the bad effects."[40] Following these principles, Magill explained Seton's situation: "The act of cooperation is justified when it occurs to achieve *a greater good or to avoid a more serious evil.*" In Seton's case, the more serious evil was the closing of the hospital and the resultant lack of health care to the poor. Specifically, "not doing good could be a serious dereliction of moral duty" by "forfeiting the valuable contribution of Brackenridge's health care to the community." The greater good was that Seton could "extend its mission and values in the community . . . , continue its provision of indigent care," protect "its witness to pro-life values, . . . and maintain and strengthen its position in the health care market."[41]

Magill emphasized that because the Daughters of Charity and Seton Medical Center did not approve of the illicit procedures or want them to take place, "there is no formal cooperation." This was also where Brackenridge's designation as a non-Catholic facility was emphasized. Even though Seton's employees would provide the sterilizations, the lease agreement stated that the city retained "reserved powers over Brackenridge." As Magill pointed out, it was very important to "clearly establish that Brackenridge is a non-Catholic hospital."[42]

The Ethics Controversy

It was the responsibility of Austin's bishop John McCarthy to approve the deal, since it involved a Catholic and non-Catholic partnership in his diocese. Considered one of the nation's more moderate bishops, McCarthy had been an activist for working men and women since the 1950s, when he became involved in the labor movement. As part of his fight for social justice, he had participated in the civil rights march in Selma, Alabama, in 1965.[43] When faced with the problem of whether or not the poor in Austin would receive care, his stance was predictable. He believed that Seton could not survive alone against the growing power of the four Columbia/HCA hospitals, which could underbid Seton for services. The hospital would then lose patients and would be forced to close.[44] Other communities cited Columbia/HCA's entry in their areas as significantly influencing their actions, as well.[45] In such a competitive environment, a partnership with Brackenridge was essential;

otherwise, the Columbia/HCA group would become the major player in the Austin hospital marketplace, which to Bishop McCarthy and the Daughters of Charity meant that the poor would not get the care they needed—one could not assume that the for-profit Columbia/HCA would provide the kind of charity care Seton had.[46] The Saint David's contract with Columbia/HCA retained the right to make some provisions for the poor, but that area was then still under negotiation. In May 1995, Bishop McCarthy wrote Sister Patricia Elder, DC, chair of Seton's board of trustees, that pending final review of the document, he supported the lease arrangement, justifying his support on the principle of material cooperation. The arrangement would maintain the Church's commitment to the poverty-stricken people of Central Texas and ensure the survival of Seton Medical Center.[47]

Despite consultation with ethicists, Catholic theologians, and other health care providers, the Seton/Brackenridge partnership triggered a long battle between the Daughters of Charity, lay Seton leaders, and Bishop McCarthy on the one hand, and the Vatican and conservative Austin laity on the other. On May 17, 1995, before the regional and national boards of the Daughters of Charity had finalized the agreement, a group calling themselves Concerned Catholics of Austin wrote to the Vatican. Using the conservative Saint Joseph Foundation in San Antonio as intermediary, they complained that the Daughters were cooperating in abortions in their hospital.[48] They addressed the letter to Joseph Cardinal Ratzinger, head of the Vatican's Congregation for the Doctrine of the Faith. This agency's role included investigating any action or publication that seemed contradictory to the faith and reproving the authors of such acts if satisfaction was not reached.[49] In June 1995, Archbishop Tarcisio Bertone, representative of the Congregation for the Doctrine of the Faith, wrote to Bishop McCarthy challenging the proposed agreement and asking the bishop not to sign the contract. In July, McCarthy aggressively defended Seton's position in writing and provided the Vatican with background information on the proposed lease. But the Vatican's response was a long time coming, arriving finally in March 1996, and meanwhile the bishop "assumed that silence meant consent"; he signed the lease in October 1995.[50]

On at least two occasions in 1997, the Vatican instructed the bishop and the Daughters of Charity to stop all sterilizations and contraceptive programs at Brackenridge. McCarthy again commissioned canon lawyers, ethicists, and health care representatives and asked for more time to study the situation. Despite all his correspondence with Vatican representatives, the bishop was unable to convince them that the city of Austin owned Brackenridge and that it was not a Catholic hospital. City officials had reserved this right and placed conditions in the agreement that reproductive services would be continued. Any breach of the contract would subject Seton to a multimillion-dollar fine. The Vatican countered that the lease agreement did not meet the tenets of Catholic moral teaching and that "formal" rather than "material" cooperation existed.[51] In June 1998, Bishop McCarthy went to Rome, where Cardinal Ratzinger asked for more detailed information about the lease. By then, the controversy was making front-page headlines in Austin.

On July 30, a story in the *Austin American Statesman* summarized the issues of the preceding three years. In it, Bishop McCarthy asserted that helping the poor was a "cornerstone of the Catholic faith. . . . We are not trying to expand our hospital empire. We don't think of health care as a business. . . . We are trying to protect health care for the poor." In the same article, Patricia Hayes, Seton's chief operating officer, highlighted Seton's commitment to the Austin community. The Daughters of Charity had hired Hayes in the late 1990s after she had served as the first woman and second lay president of Saint Edward's University for fourteen years. With a PhD in philosophy from Georgetown University, this powerful woman had vast experience in dealing with the public; she had chaired Austin's United Way and the Greater Austin Chamber of Commerce. In the article, she pointed out that in the year before the lease agreement, Seton had delivered $17 million in charity health care while the projection for the following year was close to $50 million; thus, she asserted, "Seton would never break the lease."[52]

On the day this news article appeared, Hayes wrote to Seton's board of trustees that the hospital remained in compliance with the lease agreement and that all services, including reproductive, remained available at Brackenridge. She clarified that the dialogue between Bishop McCarthy and the Vatican "was a private, internal discussion within the Church, to which Seton was not a party."[53] Similar dialogues were going on in many communities, and bishops nationwide closely watched the Austin case. The outcome could determine how much discretion they would have as more and more Catholic hospitals allied with secular facilities. An official for the Daughters of Charity National Health System noted that failure to maintain their position would influence their work with public hospitals throughout the country.[54]

An article in *The Wanderer*, a conservative Catholic publication, was scathing in its criticism of Bishop McCarthy for "deceiving" the Vatican and for presenting "a dismal portrait of episcopal solicitude for the poor and the degeneration of Catholic social teaching." Furthermore, "McCarthy showed that his view of the poor is apparently Sangerite," a reference to Margaret Sanger's advocacy for birth control.[55]

To counter this criticism, an *Austin American-Statesman* editorial on July 31, 1998, called for community support for Bishop McCarthy and provided further insight into his standoff with the Vatican: "One of the highlights of the tenure of McCarthy, a warmly regarded local leader, has been his insistence that diocesan social programs be managed at the parish level. Were the Vatican willing to confer a comparable amount of local autonomy and cease micromanaging operations at a distant hospital, a local crisis would subside."[56]

"A Wall of Separation"

If the Vatican determined that Seton did not conform to Catholic moral teaching, the hospital could lose the Church's sponsorship for its facilities. Thus through 1998, the Daughters of Charity, Bishop McCarthy, other Seton officials, and the City of Austin worked on a deal to amend the contract. In August of that year, the *Austin American-Statesman* reported that a new agreement for sterilizations and reproductive services had been negotiated that created "a wall of separation" between Seton and the services the Church deemed sinful: employees of the city-county health department would provide family-planning and counseling services, and independent practitioners, not Seton employees, would perform surgical sterilizations. Seton CEO Hayes noted that "this firewall that is important to us—and has been important from the beginning—is even stronger." To pay for the outside services, the city reduced its annual payment to Seton for indigent care at Brackenridge. This deduction from the indigent care money made it clear that Seton was not paying for city offices and services inside the hospital.[57]

Although reproductive procedures continued at Brackenridge, women's activists from Planned Parenthood and the Texas Family Planning Association, who had been consulted in the original agreement, were angry that they had not been informed of the renegotiations. "I know there is pressure from the Vatican," said the executive director of Planned Parenthood, "but once again it is this stuff behind closed doors that makes you feel very uneasy." In December 1998, the executive director of the Texas Family Planning Association stated: "I have a huge problem with the separation of church and state in this particular arrangement."[58]

The new compromise to allow city employees to do the proscribed practices remained in effect until 2001, when the USCCB revised the *Ethical and*

Religious Directives to prohibit the very solution created at Brackenridge. The move toward this revision had begun in 2000, when, with Seton's situation in the forefront, the Vatican's Congregation for the Doctrine of the Faith ordered the U.S. bishops to change the *Ethical and Religious Directives* concerning mergers and partnerships with non-Catholic facilities. Material cooperation would no longer justify sterilization and other procedures. Seton officials had remained optimistic—Hayes thought it premature to speculate on what changes might occur at Seton—but Frances Kissling of Catholics for a Free Choice (CFFC), a group based in Washington, D.C., that worked to decriminalize abortion and contraception, was more pessimistic: "As long as sterilizations take place in that building"—Seton Hospital—she had told an Austin journalist, "it is not going to pass muster with the Vatican."[59]

In 2000, Pope John Paul II appointed Bishop Gregory Aymond to succeed McCarthy on his retirement. The more conservative Aymond was known for his support of Vatican teachings, and he was the representative to the USCCB meeting in 2001 when the bishops developed the new *Ethical and Religious Directives*. They voted overwhelmingly to tighten the reins on Catholic hospitals, and their main focus was part 6 of the document, "Forming New Partnerships with Health Care Organizations and Providers." Specifically, a new Directive 70 forbade Catholic health care organizations from engaging "in immediate material cooperation in actions that are intrinsically immoral, such as abortion, euthanasia, assisted suicide, and direct sterilization."[60] According to ethicist David Kelly, this ecclesiastical decree usurped any "right use of reason" in applying principles of moral teaching. "Perhaps the intention here is to enforce a disciplinary rule in Catholic hospitals," he asserted, "rather than to suggest a change in the underlying moral teaching about material cooperation." But to Bishop Aymond, the new *Ethical and Religious Directives* provided "an opportunity to teach strongly about the respect for human life and also our belief in the sacredness of marriage and sexuality." He said he felt "very positive that the *Directives* have been clarified."[61]

Not "*If* Reproductive Services Remain Available, but *How*"

The new *Ethical and Religious Directives* forced the Daughters of Charity and Seton officials to renegotiate with the City of Austin. On June 8, 2001, Seton announced that to comply with Church teachings, they could no longer allow sterilizations and other contraceptive services to be provided at Brackenridge, even by city employees. In a press conference that day, Austin mayor Kirk Watson was adamant that reproductive services would still be available to Austin citizens, regardless of their ability to pay: "The question isn't *if* reproductive services remain available, but *how*."[62] After considering several options, the city proposed creating "a hospital within a hospital": the city would operate a separately licensed hospital on Brackenridge's fifth floor. A second entity, either the city or another health organization, would be licensed to handle the reproductive services. All sterilization and contraceptive procedures would be done on the separate floor, which also would house a labor and delivery area for low-income women who wanted ready access to sterilization when they delivered their babies, not an option in Brackenridge's labor and delivery department.[63]

Women's rights activists protested. The vice president of Austin's National Organization for Women chapter had concerns but believed that "realistically, it's the best offer we're going to get." Her organization and another women's advocacy group, the Democracy Coalition, sponsored a town hall meeting on the Brackenridge issue. Many attendees objected to a church organization running a public hospital. They planned a protest march that would start at Brackenridge and end at the Catholic Diocesan Office a few blocks away. Women's health activists did not want sterilizations moved from Brackenridge, preferring a seamless transition between a woman's delivery and her sterilization, if that was her choice. Yet a member of the Democracy Coalition noted that "moving reproductive services to a separate floor suggests something is wrong. . . . Seamlessness works great in a bra, but it does not work well in a hospital situation."[64]

A spokeswoman for the Women's Health and Family Planning Association of Texas saw this as "a discrimination issue. We're talking about low-income, uninsured women. They don't have a choice." To further complicate matters, Seton announced that emergency contraception (EC) medication would be made available to women either in its own emergency room or on the fifth floor, but only if a test proved that the woman was not ovulating at the time. Advocates for women's health wanted Brackenridge to provide the medicine to women upon request. They viewed Seton's restrictions as placing the services out of reach of the women who most needed them.[65]

Seton's actions regarding EC were in compliance with the 2001 Directive 36, which permitted Catholic hospitals to provide EC after a woman was sexually assaulted "if, after appropriate testing, there is no evidence that conception has occurred already." But Seton was in the minority in providing EC, even with restrictions, compared to other Catholic facilities. In a 1999 national survey of 589 such institutions conducted by CFFC, 82 percent said they did not provide EC at all, even if a woman had been sexually assaulted, and only 22 percent of those providing no EC gave women referrals to someone who would provide the medicine.[66]

Four more months of negotiation brought a coalition of community groups together and the compromise that resulted in the "hospital within a hospital" plan. Seton would pay for remodeling the fifth floor, which would have its own pharmacy, medical records area, nursing unit, housekeeping, and separate elevator for access. Seton also would pay approximately $500,000 less a year on its annual lease to Brackenridge; EC would be provided on the fifth floor only to women who were sexually assaulted. Seton also agreed to refer to a city clinic any woman requesting EC who had not been raped, which meant that indigent women seeking this service would not find it at the public hospital.[67] The city council approved the measure in 2002, and the Vatican had no problem with the "hospital within a hospital" system. A letter in the *Statesman* praised Seton and the Daughters of Charity: "Without Seton and its Catholic values, low-income citizens of Austin would have nowhere to turn for emergency medical treatment. . . . No organization should be condemned for following its conscience."[68]

The Daughters of Charity National Health System put Brackenridge back in the black, largely because of its many resources and its level of philanthropy; it was easier to absorb charity care across a large system. And Brackenridge continued to provide most of the city's care to the poor. According to the *Statesman*, Seton and Brackenridge together accounted for more than 60 percent of the entire system's charitable care and 80 percent of its Medicaid billings. Furthermore, millions of Medicare reimbursements went to Seton, as well as money from the city's medical assistance programs for the indigent, which its rival, Saint David's, did not get.[69]

Activists for women's reproductive rights called the 2001 *Ethical and Religious Directives* "just another example of the challenges of allowing faith-based institutions—especially the Catholic Church—to deal with public medicine."[70] In the end, however, Seton became the region's largest community service organization, home to a Level II Trauma Center, a pediatric facility, and a teaching hospital—a powerful competitor to Columbia/HCA.

The decision to create a "hospital within a hospital" system was not an easy one for the Daughters of Charity or for other Church and hospital officials, who took criticism from those on both sides of the reproductive question. Bishop McCarthy took a philosophical view of this polarization when he said, in our

2007 interview: "When the right-wing Catholics and the left-wing pro-choicers are both against you—then you know you're doing something right!"[71]

The Daughters of Charity wrestled with their collective conscience over the field of reproductive services. They were committed to care of the poor, but like all Catholic hospitals, they had to base their actions on the *Ethical and Religious Directives*. Adherence to that document was a matter of survival, as the Daughters could not afford to lose Catholic sponsorship. In the end, they responded to a hardening of the Vatican's opposition to reproductive services with an innovative compromise. It was not a case of Catholic sister nurses alone confronting hierarchical authority; rather, it involved multiple stakeholders. What the Daughters and the City of Austin especially needed to maintain their partnership, while still adhering to Catholic Church policies, was strong leadership, a clear understanding of the benefits of the partnership, and an aggressive pursuit of key goals, especially the provision of health care to all Austin's people.[72]

Cooperation and Its Limitations

After Seton and Austin signed their lease, similar collaborations involving Catholic hospitals took place in the United States, some of which were short-lived: under Vatican pressure, several had to end their agreements. In Little Rock, Arkansas, for example, the Arkansas Women's Health Center had leased space for sterilizations in a formerly secular hospital then owned by Saint Vincent Health System. After consulting the 2001 *Ethical and Religious Directives*, the Little Rock bishop directed the hospital to terminate the lease, because the Women's Health Center existed only to provide reproductive care.[73] The difference was that Brackenridge offered many services to the poor; had it existed only for reproductive care, the Daughters of Charity could not have maintained their partnership with it.

Seton's partnership differed in other ways. Ethicists from the National Catholic Bioethics Center contended that, because the circumstances of the Seton/Brackenridge partnership were unique, the revised arrangement of a "hospital within a hospital" could not be viewed as a legitimate model for other collaborative arrangements. Seton's case was "a problem of disengagement from illicit cooperation under unique circumstances." First, Brackenridge was city owned, not Catholic owned. Second, Seton was already locked into its thirty-year lease, which, if abrogated, would have caused severe consequences for its health ministry. Third, Brackenridge did need to expand its obstetric services, which were independent of the cooperation problem.

Finally, Texas law allowed licensure to be granted to two separate corporate entities operating in the same building. The city agreed to resume management of a portion of its own hospital while also promising that no abortions would be performed. The case was justifiable because of the damage not only to Seton financially if it broke the lease arrangement but also to the public that benefited from Seton's health care ministry. For any cooperation to be licit, there must be grave reason for it, which the ethicists considered to be the case with Seton and Brackenridge.[74]

Other merged facilities were unable to maintain reproductive services. According to a 1999 survey, half the mergers or partnerships between Catholic and non-Catholic hospitals resulted in the limitation or discontinuation of reproductive health services.[75] In Gilroy, California, a secular hospital merged with Saint Louise, a Catholic facility under the umbrella of Catholic Healthcare West (CHW). When CHW attempted to obtain a certificate of need to secure bond funding for a new building, antimerger activists argued that CHW did not provide adequate services because it did not offer reproductive procedures. In response, CHW mobilized local Catholics and drove them to the meeting about the certificate of need, where administrators argued that Saint Louise might not be able to remain open without the bond approval. They obtained the certificate of need, with the bishop agreeing to allow tubal ligation if a patient suffered from a medical condition that would threaten her life if she became pregnant. Other services such as emergency contraception and family-planning consultations were not retained.[76]

Writing on community activism on the issue of reproductive access in such mergers, Joyce Gelb and Colleen Shogan suggest key factors that can affect the adoption of creative solutions: the incentives for compromise, the identity of the acquiring partner in the merger, and the nature of the organized coalition that opposes the merger or partnership. In Gilroy, the secular facility exited the market, thereby increasing Saint Louise and CHW's bargaining position.[77] Other important factors include the type of association between the facilities and the local bishop's willingness to accept a creative solution. In the partnership between Seton and Brackenridge, each partner retained its separate identity; in such circumstances, some of the reproductive services in the non-Catholic hospital may be retained. Whatever the solution, the local bishop must approve it; and what one bishop may accept, another may find unacceptable.[78]

State and federal conscience clauses prohibit the government from forcing hospitals to participate in or pay for procedures they oppose on religious grounds. Yet Catholic hospital leaders sense a threat from that direction because of increasing attacks on their ability to provide services in accord with their values. Many believe that the future of Catholic health care in the United States is far from a sure thing because of the cultural divide between secular views and those of people motivated by religious convictions. James C. Capretta argues for ensuring that institutions survive that have historically built up reputations for compassion with "no other interests but the patients"—traits commonly associated with Catholic health care providers. For such a plan to become a reality, they must maintain the ability to deliver services in a way that protects their moral integrity. Right now, according to Capretta, that is uncertain.[79]

Conclusion

Supporting the Catholic Church's teachings on abortion and reproductive services became a distinct mark of Catholic hospitals' identity. With the increasing secularization of U.S. society and a growing belief in the power of science, the Vatican centralized its power. Important to this discussion is that Joseph Cardinal Ratzinger, who played such a large role in the Seton/Brackenridge controversy, is now Pope Benedict XVI.

Many assert that the negative effect of mergers on reproductive health services is small compared with the significant services Catholic hospitals provide. In 2000, the president of Pittsburgh Mercy Health System expressed disappointment that a *60 Minutes* program on Catholic health care entitled "God, Women, and Medicine" had taken a narrow view of his hospital, focusing on what it failed to provide rather than on all the services it offered. In 1999, for example, his hospital committed more than $26 million to charity and community services. Father Michael Place, president and CEO of the CHA, also protested the one-sided portrayal of Catholic health care to the show's executive producer, arguing that avoiding a procedure is not the same as imposing one's morality on others or "injecting the church into health care."[80]

Such views highlight the importance of the compromise between the Daughters of Charity and the city of Austin, because the "hospital within a hospital" solution was not possible for many Catholic hospitals. Still, the issue of provision of reproductive services caused conflict among many groups. While the Daughters found themselves at odds with the Catholic Church's newest directives proscribing such services, women's activists thought the compromise was too limited, and they accused Catholic bishops of politicizing their hospitals. Conservative Catholic advocates were unhappy that the services were offered at all. The Vatican thought that Bishop McCarthy and the Daughters were bending Church doctrine too far and initially ordered them to cease the procedures altogether. The "hospital within a hospital," however, did permit some reproductive services to continue, and it allowed the Daughters of Charity to claim that they had not abandoned their mission to the poor. To them, the outcome served as an example of their willingness to work on compromise solutions.[81] As Reverend Magill stated in the *Wall Street Journal*, if the Daughters and other Catholic providers are accused of looking for "loopholes" to allow them to maintain the status quo, "that is a risk that has to be taken."[82] The religious congregations, lay administrators, clergy, and ethicists continue to maintain a delicate balance between the Vatican's demands and their own social and religious missions within the hospital marketplace.

Chapter 8

S Stands for "Sister," Not "Stupid"

From the dawn of Catholic hospitals in America, there has existed an inherent conflict between the Church's clearly enunciated spiritual values and the market realities with which they had to compete. Over the course of the twentieth century, Catholic hospital leaders adapted to drastic market changes and to transformations within the Church that profoundly increased their moral and religious obligations to the poor and underserved. Catholic hospitals' missions to serve the needs of the most oppressed and to preserve the sacred rights of the unborn, however, often clashed head-on with practices of secular hospitals not constrained by the same moral guidelines.

Catholic sisters and brothers determined early on that if their hospitals were to survive, they would need to make at least some subtle separation between their idealistic spiritual beliefs and the practices and policies of their hospitals that, due to market forces, sometimes demanded they reduce their rigidity and dogmatism. This is not to say that Catholic sisters and brothers were hypocritical, but rather that they were pragmatic, realizing that their hospitals, in order to serve the most needy in an imperfect world, had to operate with a few imperfections of their own. This clash of spiritual ideals and market pressures has forced all Catholic hospital administrators, past and present, into a delicate dance to ensure their institutions' survival in an increasingly competitive secular marketplace without alienating their ecclesiastical elders.

There were, of course, times when they stepped out of this delicate dance. As an example, in the 1980s, when Mercy Hospital in San Diego was not being adequately reimbursed by Medicaid, Sister Felice Sauers, a Sister of Mercy and board member of the hospital, accompanied other hospital leaders to Sacramento, where they appealed to the California Health Services Committee for more money to cover their extensive Medicaid clientele. One representative on the committee commented that the hospital, being Catholic, would continue to "do good" regardless of reimbursements. Incensed at the patronizing attitude toward nuns and their work this comment revealed, Sister Felice boldly stood up and stated: "*S* stands for 'Sister,' not 'Stupid'!" The committee granted them the extra reimbursements.[1]

Sister Felice and many other sisters and brothers in Catholic health care understood that their charitable missions were inevitably strengthened or limited by their fiscal performances. In all their work, they tried never to buck the market. Without sound business models, market analyses, and trained executives, Catholic hospitals could not attract the best physicians, offer the best services, compete with other health systems, and raise the money needed for operations. Maintaining any mission to the sick and poor relied on positive financial margins.[2]

Yet a major challenge for Catholic hospitals is that, for the most part, sisters and brothers are not the face of the hospital anymore. Their influence in daily hospital operational decisions waned as governance structures moved from the religious community to lay administration and trusteeship. Professionalization and specialization have made it more difficult for some sisters and brothers to obtain positions in their hospitals. More important, their dramatically decreasing numbers have affected their hospitals' identity and led to a gap between many of the institutions' aims and the personal convictions of their lay personnel.[3] In some hospitals, the bottom line pushed charity and compassion aside. In her address to a health leadership conference in the 1970s, Sister Mary Maurita Sengelaub, RSM, then executive director of the Catholic Hospital Association (CHA), highlighted the strengths and weaknesses of Catholic hospitals. She asked how it was possible for the hospital to identify with the Church, when it was not "witnessing religious and spiritual values. . . . Is it because in many cases the institution has come to be viewed as an end in itself instead of a means to an end—service to people?"[4] By the 1990s, mergers, consolidations, and closures had eliminated many of the differences between Catholic and non-Catholic hospitals. Operating styles moved from a service-oriented approach to a corporate model.

This secularizing tendency was enhanced by the bureaucratization of health care systems, which required many layers of management and governance. With the separate incorporation of hospitals, the position of hospital administrator had to be detached from that of sister superior of the local convent. In addition, payments from Medicare and Medicaid, increasing insurance payments, and more sophisticated fund-raising activities by independent organizations made the hospital less dependent on the religious orders for financial support.[5] Persistent external forces such as governmental regulations, health maintenance organizations (HMOs), and market competition required all hospitals, both secular and religious, to bow to the relentless call for cost containment. The sisters' and brothers' free labor and their hospitals' payment of subpar salaries to nurses in earlier decades had postponed cost-containment concerns.

Thus the familiar profile of the mission-driven Catholic charity hospital began, in the last decades of the twentieth century, to face significant challenges. In 1998, Richard A. McCormick, professor of Christian ethics at the University of Notre Dame, pondered the loss of Catholic hospitals' organizational identities: "Will control by insurance companies, the spread of HMOs, and shrinking government subsidies lead to the demise of Catholic hospitals?" Many Catholic leaders were concerned that their professed mission, service to the poor, had slipped away. "The central tenet of service and care," McCormick continued, "is being diluted when the 'bottom line'—not the patient—must come first in the corporation's survival stakes." He reiterated Joseph Cardinal Bernardin's pastoral letter on health care, "A Sign of Hope," written when the cardinal was dying of cancer. Bernardin had called for a theological grounding of Catholic health care that was distinct from the aim of other hospitals: to comfort those who were suffering and give them "a reason to hope," not necessarily for a physical cure, which did not always come, but hope "rooted in God's loving care . . . that gives strength and confidence." According to the cardinal, "our primary service to those who come to us cannot be for sale." Karin Dufault, SP, also sees the importance of hope, especially within the context of human suffering, but this theological interpretation sometimes dissolves in actual practice.[6]

While sisters and brothers are less visible in their hospitals than they once were, they mentor pastoral care ministers and directors of mission effectiveness who are charged with carrying out the hospitals' original missions. These personnel provide an orientation to every new employee, during which they explain the hospital's mission; outline the rights and responsibilities of employees and patients; and delineate Catholic health care values of human dignity, the common good, sanctity of life, and stewardship of resources.[7] At Catholic

Healthcare West (CHW), for example, top leaders from the forty-two hospitals in the system, who may or may not be Catholic, participate in a rigorous three-year ministry formation program where leaders discuss the basic tenets of Catholic theology, social justice issues, good business principles, and topics such as compassion and suffering. Specific metrics such as community benefit standards are formalized in the CHW system, along with a well-integrated palliative care program, all of which reflect Catholic values. While the hospitals' Catholic identity can no longer spring from the personal presence of the sisters, other personnel try to model their hospitals' mission and values.[8]

Most important is the commitment to serve the poor, the uninsured, and the underinsured. This care not only is uncompensated but also specifically seeks out those most in need and is tailored to their special circumstances. Sister Doris Gottemoeller, RSM, first president of the Sisters of Mercy of the Americas, suggests that community health initiatives with schools, parishes, and other agencies are "not 'smart marketing,' but evidence of this commitment." Through organizing into systems, collaborating with other providers, and advocating for reform at the local and national levels, she believes, the Catholic ministry can address root causes of poverty and other ills through the commitment of resources on a broad scale.[9] This mission can be complicated, however, by controversial partnerships or mergers.

As early as 1978, Sister Mary Maurita predicted that hospital systems could maximize the influence of religious sisters and brothers who ran them, and her prediction held true for many hospitals, although as an essay in *Health Care Ethics* in 2000 noted, sometimes a Catholic partner has to shift from having "over-riding authority to [having] *influence*" if it is to carry on its ministry in a community.[10] Sister Doris describes the concept of hospital sponsorship specifically as "significant influence and ultimate control over the assets, the mission, and the quality of service of the institution."[11] Bernita McTernan, senior vice president for governance, mission integration, and philanthropy at CHW, also sees "influence" as the most appropriate descriptor; at CHW, sisters from the various congregations serve on the board of directors and have the power to appoint other board members and the CEO.[12] At other hospitals, sisters are on administrative teams as vice president of mission, and in many congregations they are on the boards of all their own order's institutions, although that is becoming more difficult as their numbers decrease.[13]

Some hospitals have kept several sisters in their facilities. One sister administrator at CHW started off with four nuns in her hospital and was able to recruit sixteen more. Most held master's degrees and positions not only in nursing but also in public health, pastoral care, and mission services. In many of the CHW facilities, sister councils meet regularly with the CEOs to exchange information. Sisters serve on boards of directors with responsibility for long-range planning and other hospital strategies. Many have the final say in selling their Catholic hospital, but not a non-Catholic hospital partner.

When the Sisters of Mercy transferred ownership of Mercy Hospital in Pittsburgh to the University of Pittsburgh Medical Center, they preserved it as a Catholic institution. It is the only Catholic hospital with specialized services in Pittsburgh. Although the sisters gave up authority over the acute care facility, they continued their influence with the poor by providing services to the most at-risk residents of the community—those facing mental illness, addictions, homelessness, abuse, and isolation.[14] Similarly, the Sisters of Providence used their influence when they transferred ownership of Providence Seattle Medical Center to Swedish Hospital. Before the sale, the sisters insured that Swedish would maintain charity care at presale levels.

As hospitals separate from their founding religious congregations, some sisters and brothers continue to be in charge of large hospitals or to serve their own congregations in positions of leadership.[15] With a bachelor's degree in medical technology and a master's degree in health facilities management, Brother Thomas Keusenkothen, CFA, has been president and CEO of Alexian Brothers Health System since 1998. He was administrator of the brothers' hospital in Boys Town, Nebraska, and other Alexian Brothers institutions and has served as a member of several boards of directors, including that of the Chicago Catholic Healthcare System.[16]

In 2005 Sister Carol Keehan, DC, was named president and CEO of the Catholic Health Association (CHA), heading its staff at offices in Washington, D.C. Sister Carol earned a bachelor of science degree in nursing from Saint Joseph's College in Emmitsburg, Maryland, and a master of science degree in business administration from the University of South Carolina. She has been board chair of Ascension Health's Sacred Heart Health System in Pensacola, Florida, and served for fifteen years as president and CEO of Providence Hospital in Washington, D.C. In 1999, the American Hospital Association recognized her with its Board of Trustees Award for her significant contributions to the association.[17] *Modern Healthcare Magazine* named Sister Carol one of the most powerful people in health care, and her renown has given her important platforms to discuss the challenges of a just health care system that expands coverage to more Americans. Another astute businesswoman who is able to blend her organizational skills with a passion for social justice is Sister Sheila

Lyne, RSM, named to Chicago's Top Ten in Health Care list in 2004. These women do not see themselves as powerful individuals but as women who share power for the common good.[18]

Sisters Sheila and Carol are nurses; indeed, Catholic hospitals have historically recognized the importance of nursing for their leadership teams. In the early twentieth century, sisters' nursing roles were considered sources of influence and prestige. Barred from the priesthood, they still could function as mediators between their patients and God.[19] Today, as they move away from the bedside into administrative and corporate roles, they use skills they learned as nurses. As Eileen Sullivan-Marx, associate dean for practice and community affairs at the University of Pennsylvania, states: "Nursing, with its emphasis on communication, problem assessment, and problem solving, is good preparation for management."[20] Sister Carol sees her role at the CHA as an opportunity to convey a personal touch to people in need across the continuum of care, another skill that nurses bring to the health care system.[21] When Sister Sheila took over the financially strapped Mercy Hospital and Medical Center in Chicago in 2001, she focused on improving the relationship between management and personnel, maintaining a personal presence by routinely walking around the hospital. She developed management retreats and seminars on what it meant to be really caring to patients. As a result, many patients who had left Mercy during its struggling years started coming back. Physicians and nurses also stayed, and the hospital benefited by their loyalty even in material ways: physicians, for example, contributed funds to replace outdated equipment.[22]

In short, Sisters Carol and Sheila addressed the challenges of a more competitive marketplace and a tightening economy not merely by crunching numbers or restructuring the hospital's workforce but also by placing greater emphasis on the human factors of hospital management. They and other sisters and brothers understood what many lay corporate managers failed to grasp: that in the business of serving people, it is people themselves that ultimately matter most—not dollars or margins or numbers, but acknowledging individuals' needs, being kind and accessible, and in short, caring more about them than about the business that serves them. To the extent that these values can prevail in modern Catholic hospitals, these hospitals' impact on U.S. medical culture will remain strong, regardless of the diminishing number of sisters and brothers who walk their halls or fill their boardrooms.

Explaining how and why many religious influences remain prominent in the hospital marketplace has been this book's focus. In the past, sociologists theorized that religion and religious ideals would lose their influence with the secularization of society. As the 1960s and 1970s brought significant changes in U.S. Catholics' lifestyles, they along with the rest of society were influenced by the growth of personal income, suburbanization, and a greater attachment to materialistic values. Bioethical issues concerning abortion and reproductive issues were becoming matters of public policy. The cultural turmoil of these years resulted in a shift away from the authority of churches. In addition, the hybrid organizational forms that emerged from the merging of Catholic and non-Catholic institutions challenged the identity of Catholic hospitals and drew the attention and concern of the Vatican. It was in this increasingly secularized environment that the Catholic Church hierarchy stepped up its influence on hospitals and health policy. Change was, once more, on the horizon.

Bishops have spoken about health care in thirteen pastoral letters, beginning in 1982. Catholic hospitals' relationships with local bishops who apply and interpret the *Ethical and Religious Directives* make them distinctive. Indeed, the 2001 revised *Ethical and Religious Directives* marked the beginning of a new and challenging chapter for Catholic hospitals as the Church hierarchy increased its presence.

Thus, rather than dying out as history has suggested, religious forces in the hospital marketplace have become transformed. Statements of the CHA and of the U.S. Conference of Catholic Bishops (USCCB) and mission statements of individual Catholic hospitals that focus on social justice, compassionate care, commitment to the poor, stewardship, universal rights to health care, and respect for the dignity of all reveal the influence of religious beliefs. So also does hospitals' adherence to Church teachings via the *Ethical and Religious Directives.*[23] Gone, however, is what Charles L. Harper and Bryan F. LeBeau label "God talk"; today Catholic hospitals focus on the language of rights and justice.[24] While these value statements support Catholic theology, the changes deemphasize Catholic dogma while stressing public inclusiveness.

At the same time, the large institutional presence of Catholic hospitals enables the Catholic Church to speak forcefully about health care issues at the policy level. Although few Catholic hospital leaders before Vatican II broke new ground in dispelling longstanding racial prejudices, driven by their commitment to social justice and spiritual ideals, today they provide bold leadership in the quest for universal health care. In addition to the work of the USCCB, the CHA has increased its visibility in the public arena by monitoring a variety of legislative and policy issues at the federal level. Every two years as a new Congress convenes, the CHA develops an advocacy agenda with input from members to target the most important issues to monitor, provides yearly policy briefs that examine the issues, and gives its position.[25]

The health care reform debates of 2009 and 2010 indicate that religion still permeates the health care system. In July 2009, the CHA published a statement calling upon legislators to enact health care reform "immediately" and joined with the American Hospital Association and Federation of American Hospitals in supporting the Obama administration's efforts to move reform forward.[26] Catholic bishops came out as a formidable force in the debate, working behind the scenes with Congress to get strong abortion restrictions inserted into both the House and Senate versions of the health care bill. The abortion-financing issue was preeminent for them and overrode their long advocacy for the poor.[27] Although the CHA did not endorse any versions of the bills, pro-life critics accused the association of going against the bishops by remaining neutral on the abortion issue. Sister Carol Keehan, as CEO and president of the CHA, assured them that the organization worked closely with the bishops. "We will compromise our preferences," she asserted, "but we will not compromise our principles." Those principles included endorsing health care that respected life from conception to a natural death.[28] Sister Carol maintained a prominent presence in the debate, attending White House events on reform and sitting in the galleries of the House and Senate as debates took place.

The CHA acknowledged the complexity of the issues, however, and was more flexible than the USCCB over certain aspects of the reform bills, particularly those that increased access to care. If universal health care was passed, hospitals that provided large amounts of uncompensated care would surely benefit, and many more people could pay their bills. Most important, those with no access to care would have access. When pressed by pro-life advocates to immediately close Catholic hospitals should abortion be accepted, Sister Carol responded with an unqualified no. Catholic health care was a critical component of the Church's ministry. "Sometimes you have to live in a very imperfect marketplace," she explained. "We *have* to be in that marketplace, standing for these issues, . . . saying this is how we take care of pregnant mothers." Most important, health reform was needed so that these mothers would have access to care. Indeed, reform would be beneficial not only because it would protect mothers and the unborn but also "the cancer patient, the person with multiple sclerosis, . . . the frail elderly and the dying person"—a strong pro-life message.[29]

Catholic hospital leaders did worry about religious liberties that could be threatened if legislation passed that infringed upon their right to uphold their own beliefs related to medical care. In 1973, for example, after abortion became legal, federal Medicaid funds could be used to pay for abortions just as for any other health service. The Hyde Amendment, however, in 1976 forbade government funding agencies to require health care providers to perform abortions and in 1977 prohibited the use of federal funds to pay for abortions. The Supreme Court upheld the constitutionality of the Hyde Amendment in 1980, and a version of it has been adopted every year since. In 1993, for instance, the Hyde Amendment permitted federal funding for abortions only if pregnancy resulted from rape or incest or if it was necessary to save the woman's life. Under the Weldon Amendment, passed in 2004, health care professionals, hospitals, health maintenance organizations, or any health insurance plan could refuse to pay for abortions, counseling, or referrals, even in cases of rape, incest, or medical emergency.[30] Yet, in some states, legislation has escalated that mandates contraception coverage in employee insurance plans that include prescription coverage. Sister Carol assured doubters that the CHA will continue to support legislative conscience clause protections.[31]

In December 2009, after many months of work on health reform legislation, an internal dispute over abortion developed among Democrats that threatened to kill reform efforts altogether. The Left advocated pro-choice abortion policies, countered by moderate Democrats who wanted to strike abortion from any benefit plan covered by the federal government. The USCCB was a key player in the debate, perhaps even the dominant one.[32] Representatives for the bishops negotiated with officials in House Speaker Nancy Pelosi's office shortly before the key vote on the health care bill in the House of Representatives. Pelosi, a Catholic, allowed abortion opponents to offer an amendment sponsored by Michigan representative Bart Stupak that prohibited any government-backed health insurance plan from funding elective abortions.[33] Abortion opponents considered it their "biggest victory in years," but the president of Planned Parenthood called it an "unconscionable power play by the Catholic bishops interceding to put their own ideology into the national health care plan."[34]

Abortion was the key negotiating issue that held up passage of a bill in the Senate as well. The bill eventually allowed any state to prohibit the use of federal subsidies for insurance plans that covered abortions and required insurers in other states to segregate subsidy money so that only funds from private premiums would cover abortions. On December 25, the *New York*

Times reported that the CHA had split with the bishops over the Senate health bill, which the USCCB called "morally unacceptable."[35] On December 28, however, Sister Carol disputed the *New York Times* report. Although it "would have made a great story," she said, "there is not a shred of disagreement between the CHA and the bishops. . . . We believe there is a great possibility and probability that in conference committee we can work toward a solution that will prevent federal funding of abortion." Emphasizing the CHA's importance in the debate, she said the CHA "brings a lot of expertise with funding structures in the marketplace" to the discussion and planned to "bring that to bear" during the conference committee's deliberations.[36]

The debate changed in January 2010, however, after the Massachusetts special election upset when voters chose Republican Scott Brown for the U.S. Senate seat formerly held by liberal Democrat Edward M. Kennedy. Even though the election altered the Democrats' so-called filibuster-proof majority in the Senate, President Barack Obama and most of the House and Senate Democrats continued their commitment to a fiscally responsible health insurance reform bill. With the bill still facing entrenched and virtually unanimous Republican opposition, Catholic sisters showed they were "still a strong force."[37] On March 3, Sister Carol was among guests invited to the White House to hear President Obama speak on health insurance reform. A week later, on March 11, the CHA sent legislators in the House of Representatives a letter signed by Sister Carol, urging them to move quickly on the representatives' plan "to enact health reform by passing the Senate-approved legislation." The CHA viewed the Senate bill as going far toward covering more than thirty million uninsured people in the country and providing needed reforms in the private insurance market while cutting the federal deficit and not providing federal funding for abortions.[38] Within hours of hearing about the CHA's action, sixty-one leaders of women's religious organizations representing 59,000 sisters joined with the CHA to support the Senate bill as written. Asserting that it would "make historic new investments—$250 million—in support of pregnant women," the sisters declared: "This is the REAL pro-life stance, and we as Catholics are all for it."[39]

With this act, thousands of sisters risked dividing themselves from the Church hierarchy, since they broke with the bishops who still opposed the bill. The USCCB statement, signed on March 15 by Francis Cardinal George of Chicago, acknowledged differences with the CHA and stated that the bill was still unclear about the abortion issue: its "flaws are so fundamental that they vitiate the good that the bill intends to promote."[40]

That sisters would take such a stand is not surprising. They were the ones who worked in the trenches with women, children, and the poor in many health care services, and they often witnessed the fatal results of denying or delaying care to those in dire need. Sisters saw the problems that developed when poor women could not get prenatal care, and the tragic misfortunes that often resulted when the sick were left alone to care for themselves.[41]

Whether by design or mere fortune, the sisters' split with Church elders over the health care bill was well timed. Catholic officials had been fighting negative public opinion over priests' sex abuse scandals for years, so the nuns' public stance in support of the bill was likely somewhat insulated from severe Church sanction. Considering their relatively low hierarchical position in relation to male Church leaders, however, the sisters' actions still could be seen as courageous and gave a degree of inspiration and political cover to some congressional members who then came out in support of the bill. Afterward, however, Sister Carol's and the other nuns' public dissent from the bishops remained a source of contention.

The historic legislation passed in the House on March 21, 2010. Revisions to the Senate bill also passed. Representative Stupak and other antiabortion Democrats held out for changes on the abortion language until President Obama agreed to sign an executive order that ensured that there would be no changes in the Hyde Amendment, which prevented federal funding for abortions. On March 23, 2010, President Obama signed the Patient Protection and Affordable Care Act (PPACA); on March 30, he signed the Health Care and Education Reconciliation Act, amending certain provisions of PPACA. Sister Carol Keehan was one of twenty people who received ceremonial pens at the signing.

The support of the Catholic Church's teaching on abortion and reproductive services is one example of how religious beliefs continue to affect hospital policy and modern health care and also reveals the conflicts within the Church over how much to pit opposition to abortion and other procedures against concerns for social justice.[42] All the problems and possibilities noted here reflect gray areas of Catholic health care at the end of the twentieth century. They also provoke further questions. For example, can religious groups that receive federal money for social services perform only those procedures that conform to their faith? (Catholic health care leaders answer a resounding yes.) When the government imposes mandates for not-for-profit hospitals to meet charity requirements, do health policies support hospitals' abilities to do so?

Another question involves the Vatican's relationship with the U.S. sisters, whose religious lives, even before the health reform debate, were facing greater scrutiny. In 2009, the Vatican began a three-year investigation of the women's religious congregations and requested they answer a questionnaire that the sisters found offensive. Consequently, the vast majority did not comply. Some nuns feared the Church was trying to reestablish traditional convent standards, when sisters wore distinct habits and organized their workdays around specific prayer schedules. Others voiced concerns that the Vatican was investigating whether sisters had strayed too far from Church teachings. The Church's investigation provided further fuel for critics of Pope Benedict XVI, who charged he was supporting traditionalists hostile to Vatican II reforms.[43]

Challenges like these await Catholic hospitals in the twenty-first century as they strive to be religious institutions in a secular society.

Notes

Archives frequently cited in the notes have been identified by the following abbreviations:

ABA   Alexian Brothers Provincial Archives, Arlington Heights, Illinois
ADOC   Marillac Provincial House Archives of the Daughters of Charity, St. Louis, Missouri
AHC   Austin History Center, Austin, Texas
ASM   Sisters of Mercy of the Americas West Midwest–Chicago Community Archives, Chicago
ASSJR   Archives, Sisters of St. Joseph, Rochester, New York
CAT   Catholic Archives of Texas, Austin
CHM   Chicago Historical Museum
MHA   Mercy Hospital Archives, Chicago
PHO   Providence Hospital, Oakland, California Collection, SPA
PSMC   Providence Seattle Medical Center Collection, SPA
RPP   Sister John Gabriel Ryan Personal Papers Collection, SPA
SMA   Sisters of Mercy Archives, Chicago
SPA   Sisters of Providence Archives, Mother Joseph Province, Seattle
UPMC   Mercy Archives University of Pittsburgh Medical Center/Mercy Hospital Archives, Pittsburgh

Chapter 1 — From Sisters in Habits to Men in Suits

1. Although the word "nun" specifically refers to a member of a cloistered religious order, I use it interchangeably throughout this book with "sister" and "women religious." For books on sisters and hospitals, see Sioban Nelson, *Say Little, Do Much: Nursing, Nuns, and Hospitals in the Nineteenth Century* (Philadelphia: University of Pennsylvania Press, 2001); Bernadette McCauley, *Who Shall Take Care of Our Sick? Roman Catholic Sisters and the Development of Catholic Hospitals in New York City* (Baltimore: Johns Hopkins University Press, 2005).

2. Patricia Wittberg, *From Piety to Professionalism—and Back? Transformations of Organized Religious Virtuosity* (Lanham, Md.: Lexington Books, 2006).

3. Philip Gleason, *Speaking of Diversity: Language and Ethnicity in Twentieth-Century America* (Baltimore: Johns Hopkins University Press, 1992), 295.

4. Charles R. Morris, *American Catholic: The Saints and Sinners Who Built America's Most Powerful Church* (New York: Vintage Books, 1997), 254. See also R. Scott Appleby, "Decline or Relocation? The Catholic Presence in Church and Society, 1950–2000," in *The Church Confronts Modernity: Catholicism since 1950 in the U.S., Ireland, and Quebec,* ed. Leslie Woodcock Tentler (Washington, D.C.: Catholic University of America Press, 2007), 235.

5. MergerWatch, "Religious Health Restrictions Threaten Women's Health and Endanger Women's Lives," September 2004.

6. *The Official Catholic Directory* (New York: P. J. Kenedy and Sons, 2008).

7. Barbra Mann Wall, *Unlikely Entrepreneurs: Catholic Sisters and the Hospital Marketplace, 1865–1925* (Columbus: Ohio State University Press, 2005).
8. Stephen M. Shortell, "The Evolution of Hospital Systems: Unfulfilled Promises and Self-Fulfilling Prophesies," *Medical Care Review* 45, no. 2 (Fall 1988): 178.
9. Center for Applied Research in the Apostolate, "Frequently Requested Catholic Church Statistics," http://cara.georgetown.edu/bulletin/index.htm. Accessed December 8, 2009. See also Sandra M. Schneiders, "Why They Stayed," *National Catholic Reporter*, August 17, 2009, http://ncronline.org/news/women/why-they-stayed. Accessed December 8, 2009.
10. *The Official Catholic Directory*, 1960 and 1990.
11. Arthur Jones, "Huge Nonprofit System Feels Pressure to Cut Costs, Merge, and Get Bigger," *National Catholic Reporter*, June 16, 1995, 11–15; Center for Applied Research in the Apostolate, "Frequently Requested Catholic Church Statistics."
12. "Religious Personnel," 1960, 1986, 1990, (56) PSMC, History, SPA. Currently, the chair of the board of directors is a layperson.
13. Christopher J. Kauffman, *The Ministry of Healing*, vol. 2 of *The History of the Alexian Brothers* (New York: Seabury Press, 1978).
14. Monica Langley, "Money Order: Nuns' Zeal for Profits Shapes Hospital Chain, Wins Wall Street Fans," *Wall Street Journal*, January 7, 1998.
15. Rosemary Stevens, *In Sickness and in Wealth: American Hospitals in the Twentieth Century* (Baltimore: Johns Hopkins University Press, 1989; repr. 1999).
16. Wittberg, *From Piety to Professionalism*; C. A. Hangartner, "Implications for Nursing Education from Vatican II," *Hospital Progress* 47 (October 1966): 63–33, 78.
17. Stevens, *In Sickness and in Wealth*, 339.
18. Wittberg, *From Piety to Professionalism*; Lee Clarke and Carroll L. Estes, "Sociological and Economic Theories of Markets and Nonprofits: Evidence from Home Health Organizations," *American Journal of Sociology* 97, no. 4 (January 1992): 945–969; Mary Ruggie, "The Paradox of Liberal Intervention: Health Policy and the American Welfare State," *American Journal of Sociology* 97, no. 4 (January 1992): 919–944; Mary L. Fennell and Jeffrey A. Alexander, "Perspectives on Organizational Change in the US Medical Care Sector," *Annual Review of Sociology* 19 (1993): 89–112.
19. Peter L. Berger, *The Sacred Canopy: Elements of a Sociological Theory of Religion* (New York: Doubleday, 1967); Linda Woodhead, ed., *Peter Berger and the Study of Religion* (New York: Routledge, 2001).
20. James A. Morone, *Hellfire Nation: The Politics of Sin in American History* (New Haven: Yale University Press, 2003); Christian Smith, *The Secular Revolution: Power, Interests, and Conflict in the Secularization of American Public Life* (Berkeley: University of California Press, 2003); David Martin, *On Secularization: Towards a Revised General Theory* (Burlington, Vt.: Ashgate, 2005); Charles Taylor, *A Secular Age* (Cambridge, Mass.: Belknap Press, 2007); and Peter Berger, Grace Davie, and Effie Fokas, *Religious America, Secular Europe? A Theme and Variations* (Burlington, Vt.: Ashgate, 2008). For an analysis of the persistence of religion among African American women, see Anthea D. Butler, *Women in the Church of God in Christ: Making a Sanctified World* (Chapel Hill: University of North Carolina Press, 2007).
21. Karel Dobbelaere, *Secularization: An Analysis at Three Levels* (New York: P.I.E. Peter Lang, 2002), 35 (emphasis in original).

22. Daniel Callahan and Angela A. Wasunna, *Medicine and the Market: Equity v. Choice* (Baltimore: Johns Hopkins University Press, 2006); David F. Kelly, *Contemporary Catholic Health Care Ethics* (Washington, D.C.: Georgetown University Press, 2004); Leslie Woodcock Tentler, ed., *The Church Confronts Modernity: Catholicism since 1950 in the U.S., Ireland, and Quebec* (Washington, D.C.: Catholic University of America Press, 2007).

23. Charles E. Rosenberg, *Our Present Complaint* (Baltimore: Johns Hopkins University Press, 2007).

24. Paul Starr, *The Social Transformation of American Medicine* (New York: Basic Books, 1982); Kristin Luker, *Abortion and the Politics of Motherhood* (Berkeley: University of California Press, 1984); Leslie Reagan, *When Abortion Was a Crime: Women, Medicine, and Law in the U.S., 1867–1973* (Berkeley: University of California Press, 1998); Ellen Carol Dubois and Lynn Dumenil, *Through Women's Eyes: An American History with Documents* (Boston: Bedford/St. Martin's, 2005).

25. Thomas C. Fox, "Women Religious Not Complying with Vatican Study," *National Catholic Reporter*, n.d., http://ncronline.org/pring/15950. Accessed December 18, 2009.

26. Kenneth Briggs, *Double Crossed: Uncovering the Catholic Church's Betrayal of American Nuns* (New York: Doubleday, 2006).

27. Patricia Byrne, "A Tumultuous Decade, 1960–1970," in *Transforming Parish Ministry: The Changing Roles of Catholic Clergy, Laity, and Women Religious*, ed. Jay P. Dolan, R. Scott Appleby, Patricia Byrne, and Debra Campbell (New York: Crossroad, 1990), 154–175.

28. Patricia Byrne, "Diminishment, Disillusion, Discovery, 1970," in ibid., 188; Karen M. Kennelly, CSJ, *The Religious Formation Conference, 1954–2004* (Silver Spring, Md.: Religious Formation Conference, 2009).

29. Christopher J. Kauffman, *A Commitment to Healthcare: Celebrating 75 Years of the Catholic Health Association* (St. Louis: Catholic Health Association, 1990), 38; Sister M. Charles Borromeo, ed., *The New Nuns* (New York: New American Library, 1967); Marjorie Noterman Beane, *From Framework to Freedom: A History of the Sister Formation Conference* (Lanham, Md.: University Press of America, 1993); Kennelly, *The Religious Formation Conference;* Sister Formation Conference/Religious Formation Conference Records, 1936–, Department of Special Collections and University Archives, Raynor Memorial Libraries, Marquette University, http://www.marquette.edu/library/collections/archives/Mss/SFC/mss-sfc%20scope-content.htm. Accessed November 15, 2009.

30. Byrne, "A Tumultuous Decade."

31. Maureen Sullivan, *The Road to Vatican II: Key Changes in Theology* (New York: Paulist Press, 2007), 120. See also http://en.wikipedia.org/wiki/Aggiornamento. Accessed December 5, 2009.

32. John T. McGreevy, *Catholicism and American Freedom: A History* (New York: W. W. Norton, 2003).

33. Fox, "Women Religious Not Complying."

34. Meeting of the General Council, Archives of the Sisters of Saint Joseph, Rochester, N.Y.

35. Ibid.; Jay P. Dolan, *In Search of an American Catholicism: A History of Religion and Culture in Tension* (New York: Oxford University Press, 2002); McGreevy,

Catholicism and American Freedom; Michael Dominic W. Ledoux, "Decline of Religious Life: A Success Story," *Review for Religious,* March–April 2002, 183–190.

36. Dolan, *In Search of an American Catholicism.*

37. Wall, *Unlikely Entrepreneurs*; History Online, http://www2.providence.org/phs/archives/history-online/Pages/default.aspx. Accessed September 11, 2008.

38. Nelson, *Say Little, Do Much.*

39. I. Wiegers, "History of the Aachen Alexian Brothers, Aachen, Germany," ABA; Kauffman, *The Ministry of Healing*; Lawrence Davidson, *The Alexian Brothers of Chicago: An Evolutionary Look at the Monastery and Modern Health Care* (New York: Vantage Press, 1990).

40. Elizabeth Rapley, *The Devotes: Women and Church in Seventeenth-Century France* (Montreal: McGill-Queen's University Press, 1990).

41. The Emmitsburg sisters first began staffing hospitals in the continental United States in 1823 at the Baltimore Infirmary. Sister Daniel Hannefin, *Daughters of the Church: A Popular History of the Daughters of Charity in the United States, 1809–1987* (Brooklyn, N.Y.: New City Press, 1989). Elizabeth Ann Seton was canonized by Pope Paul VI in 1975, the first native-born U.S. citizen to be canonized.

42. Sister M. Cornelius Meerwald, *History of the Pittsburgh Mercy Hospital, 1847–1959* (Pittsburgh: Sisters of Mercy, 1959).

43. Commission on Hospital Care, *Hospital Care in the United States* (New York: Commonwealth Fund, 1947), 52, 65; Charles E. Rosenberg, *The Care of Strangers* (Baltimore: Johns Hopkins University Press, 1987).

44. Commission on Hospital Care, *Hospital Care in the United States*, 53–55; Stevens, *In Sickness and in Wealth.*

45. "Catholic Hospitals Plan Wide Expansion," *New York Times,* June 19, 1946. The Catholic Hospital Association became the Catholic Health Association in 1979.

46. Stevens, *In Sickness and in Wealth*, 259.

47. *The Official Catholic Directory* (New York: P. J. Kenedy and Sons, 1945–2000).

48. Rosemary Stevens, "Medicare and the Transformation of the Medical Economy," in *Major Problems in the History of American Medicine and Public Health,* ed. John Harley Warner and Janet A. Tighe (Boston: Houghton Mifflin, 2001), 487; Ronald L. Numbers, "The Third Party: Health Insurance in America," in *The Therapeutic Revolution: Essays in the Social History of American Medicine,* ed. Morris J. Vogel and Charles E. Rosenberg (Philadelphia: University of Pennsylvania Press, 1979), 177–200.

49. Joy Clough, *In Service to Chicago: The History of Mercy Hospital* (Chicago: Mercy Hospital and Medical Center, 1979); "Contemporary Needs in the Formation of the Sister for Hospital Work," *Little Journal of Providence,* May 1960, Sisters of Providence Schools of Nursing Collection, Box 1, History/Guidelines, SPA.

50. Kauffman, *A Commitment to Healthcare,* 38; Borromeo, *The New Nuns*; Beane, *From Framework to Freedom*; Historical Note, http://www.marquette.edu/library/collections/archives/Mss/SFC/mss-sfc%20scope-content.htm. Accessed November 15, 2009.

51. Conversations on Ministry: Sister Karin Dufault, http://www.sistersofprovidence.net/conversations-dufault.php. Accessed February 16, 2009. Sister Karin Dufault held several high administrative positions, and in 2008, she was vice president of mission leadership of Providence Health System.

52. Kauffman, *The Ministry of Healing*; Brothers Sebastian Brogan and John Black-ledge, *Diary of the Alexian Brothers School of Nurses*, ABA.

53. "Contemporary Needs"; "Seattle University School of Nursing, 1951–1952," PSMC, Box 52, School of Nursing, SPA.

54. "Seton Infirmary," *Austin American-Statesman*, July 19, 1936, AF—Hospitals—Seton H2770 (1), AHC; Hannefin, *Daughters of the Church*, 179; Sister Betty Ann McNeil, D.C., Archivist for the Daughters of Charity, Emmitsburg, Md., e-mail communication, May 12, 2009.

55. Local Superior to Mother Mary Barnardine, 1938, *1951 Annual Report*, Mercy Hospital, Chicago, Illinois, SMA. See also *1952 Annual Report, Mercy Hospital*, MHA; and Clough, *In Service to Chicago*.

56. Roberta Mayhew West, *History of Nursing in Pennsylvania* (Harrisburg, Pa.: Evan-gelical Press, 1939); Meerwald, *History of the Pittsburgh Mercy Hospital*; Sister Jerome McHale, *On the Wing: The Story of the Pittsburgh Sisters of Mercy, 1843–1968* (New York: Seabury Press, 1980); *Pillar of Pittsburgh: The History of Mercy Hospital and the City It Serves* (Pittsburgh: Sisters of Mercy, n.d.).

57. Joan E. Lynaugh and Barbara L. Brush, *American Nursing: From Hospitals to Health Systems* (Malden, Mass.: Blackwell, 1996), 46.

58. "The Nation's Hospitals: A Statistical Profile," Part 2, *Hospital Statistics* 45, (August 1, 1971): 447.

59. Julie Fairman and Joan E. Lynaugh, *Critical Care Nursing: A History* (Philadel-phia: University of Pennsylvania Press, 2000).

60. Stevens, *In Sickness and in Wealth*, 294.

61. "His First Impression of Mercy Hospital—The Admitting Process!" *Footnotes of Mercy Hospital and Medical Center*, Chicago, Illinois, Fall 1975, MHA.

62. Stevens, "Medicare and the Transformation," 286–287, 323; Phil Rheinecker, "Catholic Healthcare Enters a New World," in *A Commitment to Healthcare*, ed. Kauffman, 44; Mike Brennan, "Hospitals Competed in Changing Times," *Everett Herald*, August 15, 1993; John K. Iglehart, "Where Money and Medicine Meet: A Conversation with HCFA Administrator Carolyne K. Davis," *Health Affairs* 4, no. 2 (Summer 1985): 72–81.

63. Harry A. Sultz and Kristina M. Young, *Health Care USA: Understanding Its Orga-nization and Delivery* (Sudbury, Mass.: Jones and Bartlett, 2006); AHA Workforce Survey Results, June 2001, TrendWatch Chartbook 2000 (the Lewin Group).

64. Thomas R. Prince and Ramachandran Ramanan, "Operating Performance and Financial Constraints of Catholic Community Hospitals, 1986–1989," *Health Care Management Review* 19, no. 4 (1994): 38–48.

65. M. Brown, P. R. Donnelly, and D. Warner, "The Growing Multihospital System: A Sleeping Giant Stirs," *Hospital Progress* 61 (December 1980): 36–42.

66. Sister Mary Maurita Sengelaub, "Catholic Health Care Systems: A Sign of the Times," *Hospital Progress* 59, no. 11 (November 1978): 52–56.

67. Ibid.

68. Sister Helene Lentz, e-mail to author, November 5 and December 9, 2009. Sis-ter Helene is a member of the Congregation of Saint Joseph and has served as vice president for mission in various hospitals. She currently is on the Ascension Health Sponsor Council.

69. Shortell, "The Evolution of Hospital Systems"; Arthur Jones, "Catholic Aim: Aid Poor, Survive," *National Catholic Reporter*, June 6, 2003, 3–4; Alan M. Zuckerman

and Russell C. Coile, "Catholic Healthcare's Future," *Health Progress* 78, no. 6 (November–December 1997), http://www.chausa.org/Pub/MainNav/News/HP/ Archive/1997/11NovDec/Articles/Special. Accessed December 30, 2007.

70. John K. Iglehart, "Hospitals, Public Policy, and the Future: An Interview with John Alexander McMahon," *Health Affairs* 3, no. 3 (Fall 1984): 24.

71. Ursula Stepsis and Dolores Liptak, eds., *Pioneer Healers: The History of Women Religious in American Health Care* (New York: Crossroad, 1989).

72. "72nd Annual Catholic Health Assembly," *Health Progress* 68, no. 4 (July–August 1987): 66–87.

73. Kathleen Levit, Mark S. Freeland, and Daniel R. Waldo, "Data Watch—National Health Care Spending Trends: 1988," *Health Affairs* 9, no. 2 (Summer 1990): 171.

74. Stephen Zuckerman, Gloria Bazzoli, Amy Davidoff, and Anthony LoSasso, "How Did Safety-Net Hospitals Cope in the 1990s?" *Health Affairs* 20, no. 4 (July–August 2001): 159.

75. Jones, "Huge Nonprofit System," 12.

76. Peter J. Cunningham and Ha T. Tu, "A Changing Picture of Uncompensated Care," *Health Affairs* 16, no. 4 (July–August 1997): 167–175; Graham Atkinson, W. David Helms, and Jack Needleman, "State Trends in Hospital Uncompensated Care," *Health Affairs* 16, no. 4 (July–August 1997): 233–241.

77. Bruce C. Vladeck, "Paying for Hospitals' Community Service," *Health Affairs* 25, no. 1 (January–February 2006): 34–43; Allen Dobson, Joan DaVanzo, and Namrata Sen, "The Cost-Shift Payment 'Hydraulic': Foundation, History, and Implications," *Health Affairs* 25, no. 1 (January–February 2006): 22–33.

78. Vladeck, "Paying for Hospitals' Community Service"; Dobson, DaVanzo, and Sen, "The Cost-Shift Payment 'Hydraulic.'"

79. *1995 Annual Survey of Hospitals* (Chicago: American Historical Association, 1996).

80. Ibid.

81. Dobson et al., "The Cost-Shift"; Dana Beth Weinberg, *Code Green: Money-Driven Hospitals and the Dismantling of Nursing* (Ithaca, N.Y.: Cornell University Press, 2003).

82. Glenn Melnick, Emmett Keeler, and Zack Zwanziger, "Market Power and Hospital Pricing: Are Nonprofits Different?" *Health Affairs* 18, no. 3 (May–June 1999): 167–173.

83. Dobson et al., "The Cost-Shift"; "Health Care Inflation Revives in Minneapolis Despite Cost-Cutting," *Wall Street Journal*, May 19, 1998.

84. The Clayton Antitrust Act passed in 1914, and the Federal Trade Commission was established to enforce the act. See *Hospital Corp. of America v. FTC*, 807 F.2d 1381, 1386 (7th Cir. 1986, *cert. denied*, 481 U.S. 1038 [1987]). For information on this and more on antitrust enforcement and hospital mergers, see http://www.ftc.gov/bc/ hmerg1.shtm. Accessed November 20, 2009.

Chapter 2 — A Precarious Economic Scene

1. *Providence Seattle Medical Center, Seattle, WA. Chronicles*, (56), PSMC, Box 1, History, SPA.

2. For a good review of nursing and general hospitals, see Charles Rosenberg, *The Care of Strangers: The Rise of America's Hospital System* (Baltimore: Johns Hopkins University Press, 1987); and Joan Lynaugh, "Nursing's History: Looking

Backward and Seeing Forward," in *Enduring Issues in American Nursing*, ed. Ellen D. Baer, Patricia D'Antonio, Sylvia Rinker, and Loan E. Lynaugh (New York: Springer, 2001). For histories of religious hospitals, see Christopher Kauffman, *Ministry and Meaning: A Religious History of Catholic Health Care in the United States* (New York: Crossroad, 1995); Alan M. Kraut and Deborah A. Kraut, *Covenant of Care: Newark Beth Israel and the Jewish Hospital in America* (New Brunswick, N.J.: Rutgers University Press, 2007); and Guenter B. Risse, *Mending Bodies, Saving Souls: A History of Hospitals* (New York: Oxford University Press, 1999).

3. *1995 Annual Survey of Hospitals* (Chicago: American Historical Association, 1996); Rosemary Stevens, *In Sickness and in Wealth: American Hospitals in the Twentieth Century* (Baltimore: Johns Hopkins University Press, 1989; repr. 1999).

4. *Chronicles*, June 3, 1942, and 1967, PSMC, SPA.

5. "Increase in Open Heart Surgery," 1973; "Providence Foundation of Seattle," "Hospice," "Joint Commission," and "Phase I Construction," 1979; and "Providence Foundation, 1988," all in PSMC, History; *Providence Medical Center Annual Report*, 1982, SPA.

6. *Chronicles*, 1988–1989, PSMC, History. 7. "Summary," *Chronicles*, 1982 and 1983; "Charity Care," 1983, "Pacific Medical Center," 1987, "Providence Foundation," 1988, "Summary," 1992, all in PSMC, History.

8. Daniel Callahan and Angela A. Wasunna, *Medicine and the Market: Equity v. Choice* (Baltimore: Johns Hopkins University Press, 2006).

9. "Annual Ethics Conference," 1986, PSMC, SPA.

10. Barbra Mann Wall, *Unlikely Entrepreneurs: Catholic Sisters and the Hospital Marketplace, 1865–1925* (Columbus: Ohio State University Press, 2005).

11. "Introduction," and "Quality of Worklife Survey Results," 1987, PSMC, SPA.

12. See "Legislative Issues; "Mission Effectiveness Conferences"; "Medical Staff Annual Retreat," 1992; "Reorganization," 1995, PSMC, SPA.

13. "Religious Personnel," 1990, 1991, 2000, (56), PSMC, History, SPA.

14. "Leadership," 1991; "Summary, 1992"; "Fiscal Update," 1992, PSMC, SPA.

15. "Leadership," 1991, PSMC, SPA.

16. Ibid. See also Tom Paulson, "Swedish Hospital Buying Rival Providence," *Seattle Post-Intelligencer*, March 1, 2000.

17. "Fiscal Update," 1993, SPA; Paulson, "Swedish Hospital"; Pamela A. Paul-Shaheen, "The States and Health Care Reform: The Road Traveled and Lessons Learned from Seven That Took the Lead," *Journal of Health Politics, Policy, and Law* 23, no. 2 (April 1998): 319–361. In 1995, the sisters changed the facility's name to Providence Seattle Medical Center.

18. *Chronicles*, 2000; Paulson, "Swedish Hospital."

19. Information in this paragraph came from *Chronicles of the Sisters of Providence* for the years 1990–2000. See also *Board Bulletin*, System Office Publications (February 2000), SPA.

20. Memorandum to Sisters of Providence from Sister Barbara Schamber, SP, and Sister Karin Dufault, SP, re. Strategic Alliance with Swedish Health System, February 29, 2000, PSMC, History—Alliance with Swedish, 2000, SPA; Tyrone Beason, "Economics of Hospital Merger," Seattle Edition, *Seattle Times*, March 1, 2000 ; Kim Barker and Tyrone Beason, "Swedish, Providence Join," *Seattle Times*, February 20, 2000; "Swedish Gets OK to Acquire Providence," *Seattle Times*, July 20, 2000.

21. Beason, "Economics of Hospital Merger."

22. Paulson, "Swedish Hospital."

23. Karin Dufault to Sisters of Providence, August 12, 1993, Providence Everett Medical Center, Merger, 1993–1994, SPA; Mike Brennan, "Hospitals Competed in Changing Times," and "General and Providence Hospital History," *Everett Herald*, August 15, 1993; Sharon J. Salyer, "Anatomy of a Merger," *Everett Herald*, August 15, 1993; Phil Rheinecker, "Community Support Facilitates Merger," *Health Progress* 75, no. 7 (September 1994), http://www.chausa.org/PUb/MainNav/News/HP/Archive/1994/09Sept/Columns/hp9409i. Accessed December 30, 2007.

24. Sisters of Providence Health System, *Board Bulletin*, February 2000 and Summer 2000, System Office Publications, Box 4; Karin Dufault to Sisters of Providence, August 12, 1993; Sharon J. Slayer, "Everett Hospitals to Merge," August 13, 1993, *Everett Herald*; "Providence Health System to Sell Yakima and Toppenish Hospitals and Homecare to Health Management Associates," news release, March 19, 2003; and Memorandum to Board of Directors and Committee Members from Hank Walker and John Koster, "News Regarding Central Washington Service Area," all in (80) Providence Health and Services, Central Washington Service Area Sale to HMA, 2003, SPA.

25. Sister Karin Dufault, SP, RN, PhD, "Testimony, The Special Committee on Aging Hearing: Mandatory or Optional? The Truth about Medicaid," http://aging.senate.gov/events/hr144kd.pdf. Accessed November 20, 2009.

26. Eldercare, http://www.seniorjournal.com/NEWS/Eldercare/2–08–08PACE.htm. Accessed June 7, 2009. PACE is a fully capitated managed care program in which the Centers for Medicare and Medicaid Services pay the Medicare capitation and each state pays the Medicaid capitation.

27. Stevens, *In Sickness and in Wealth*, 315.

28. John T. McGreevy, *Parish Boundaries: The Catholic Encounter with Race in the Twentieth-Century Urban North* (Chicago: University of Chicago Press, 1996).

29. Jay P. Dolan, *The American Catholic Experience: A History of Colonial Times to the Present* (Notre Dame, Ind.: University of Notre Dame Press, 1992).

30. *61st Annual Report, 1926; 85th Annual Report*, 1950; and *95th Annual Report, 1960*, ABA.

31. Alexian Brothers Hospital, Chicago, Illinois, Balance Sheet for 1940, ABA.

32. Lawrence Davidson, *The Alexian Brothers of Chicago: An Evolutionary Look at the Monastery and Modern Health Care* (New York: Vantage Press, 1990).

33. Donald Dewey, *Where the Doctors Have Gone* (Chicago: Chicago Regional Hospital Study, Illinois Regional Medical Program, 1973); Kenneth T. Jackson, *Crabgrass Frontier: The Suburbanization of the United States* (New York: Oxford University Press, 1985); Douglas S. Massey and Nancy A. Denton, *American Apartheid: Segregation and the Making of the Underclass* (Cambridge, Mass.: Harvard University Press, 1993).

34. Chicago Community Planning Meeting, May 25, 1959; June 7, 1959; January 22, 1961; and February 1, 1961, ABA; Brother Gregory to Brother Fidelis, November 6, 1961, all in ABA.

35. Brother Flavian to Brother Provincial, February 27, 1961, and Planning Committee Report, 1961, both in ABA; Davidson, *The Alexian Brothers of Chicago*; Congregation of Alexian Brothers History, http://www.alexianbrothers.org/index.php?src=directoryandview=historyandsubmenu=historyandrefno=13andsrctype=history_detail. Accessed February 24, 2009.

36. Chicago Hospital Council, *Bulletin* 25, no. 2 (February 1962); "Women to Get Floor at 'Men Only' Hospital," *Chicago Tribune*, February 2, 1962. See also Chicago Planning Committee, November 5, 1961, ABA.

37. Herman Smith Consultants, "Report: Future of Alexian Brothers Hospital," June 1968; and Opinion Poll, July 1968, both in ABA.

38. "Statement by Brother Flavian Renaud, CFA, at Press Conference July 18, 1968; and Brother Flavian Renaud to Archbishop John Cardinal Cody, July 11, 1978, both in ABA. The provincial provides leadership to the brothers of the province. He is concerned with the spiritual and apostolic role of those he leads, and he leads the Provincial Council in carrying out its duties. See "Alexian Brothers Way of Life," ABA.

39. Davidson, *The Alexian Brothers of Chicago.*

40. *The Alexian Report, 1975*, ABA.

41. Marshall Bennett, Chair Board of Trustees, to Doctors, October 27, 1971, ABA. See also "New Bylaws at Alexian Brothers MC, Elk Grove, Ill., Recognize Board's Final Responsibility," *Washington News Report*, April 1973; "Medical Staff Bylaws Revision Stirs Controversy," *Trustee* 26, no. 6 (June 1973): 6; Arthur Owens, "Will Your Hospital Soon Hold All the Cards?" *Medical Economics* (December 10, 1973): 128–151.

42. "Landmark Public Health Laws and Court Decisions," *Encyclopedia of Public Health*, http://www.answers.com/topic/landmark-public-health-laws-and-court-decisions?cat=health. Accessed May 14, 2008; "Special Report: American Medical Association Annual Meeting," *Hospitals, JAHA* 47 (August 1, 1973): 26a–26d. *Bing v. Thunig* was another important decision that put responsibility for the quality of hospital service on the hospitals themselves. See Stevens, *In Sickness and in Wealth.*

43. Judy Nicol, "Alexian Brothers Case Points Up Issue of Doctor's Role," *Chicago Sun Times*, March 19, 1973; "Illinois MDs Seek Strong Role for Medical Staff," *American Medical News*, April 19, 1973, n.p.

44. "Special Report: American Medical Association Annual Meeting."

45. "Doctors Join Staff Because of Alexian Brothers' New Bylaws," *Up-To-Date* 24, no. 33 (August 27, 1973): 1; James R. Slawny to Don Kessler (Joint Commission on Accreditation of Hospitals), June 20, 1973, copy in Owens, "Will Your Hospital Soon Hold All the Cards?"

46. "Alexian Brothers Medical Center," in Msgr. Harry C. Koenig, *Institutional History of the Archdiocese of Chicago* (Caritas Christi Urget, 1981).

47. Metropolitan Chicago Healthcare Council, "The Changing Face of Health Care: Competition Heats Up," June 6, 1986, ABA; Congregation of Alexian Brothers History, http://www.alexianbrothers.org/index.php?src=directoryandview=history andsubmenu=historyandrefno=13andsrctype=history_detail. Accessed February 24, 2009.

48. Council Meeting, December 13, 1985, ABA; Johanna Stoyva, "Opposition to AIDS Bills Escalates; Veto Campaign Underway," *Outlines*, July 2, 1987.

49. This venture was in collaboration with the Archdiocese of Chicago. My thanks to Donna Dahl, archivist, for her help with this topic. See also Congregation of Alexian Brothers History, http://www.alexianbrothers.org/index.php?src=directory andview=historyandsubmenu=historyandrefno=21andsrctype=history_detail. Accessed February 21, 2009.

50. Jerry Crimmins, "Hospital Plans Takeover of Troubled Mental Health Center," *Chicago Tribune*, October 26, 1996; Diana Wallace and Chrystal Caruthers, "Alexian Acquires Hoffman Estates Medical Center," *Chicago Daily Herald*, August 20, 1998. See also Congregation of Alexian Brothers History, http://www.alexian brothers.org/index.php?src=directoryandview=historyandsrctype=detailandref no=28andcategory=History. Accessed April 10, 2009.

51. Congregation of Alexian Brothers History, http://www.bonaventurehouse.org/. Accessed November 3, 2009.

52. "A Rich Tradition of Caring for the Poor," *Seton Heartbeat* 3, no. 2 (February 28, 1996), n.p. See also "The Daughters of Charity," n.d., CAT; and Daughters of Charity, St. Vincent's Health System, http://www.stvhs.com/healthsystem/daughters .asp. Accessed February 15, 2009.

53. Central Texas—History and Heritage—About Seton, http://www.seton.net/about _seton/setons_history_and_heritage/central_texas. Accessed September 11, 2008. See also "A Tradition of Excellence: The Growth of Seton from Infirmary to Hospital to Medical Center," AF Hospitals, H2770 (1)/General, ADOC.

54. See "Open House Will Pay Tribute to Sisters," *Austin American-Statesman*, February 21, 1954; $1 Million Seton Wing Open for Public Today," copy in AF—Hospitals—Seton H2770 (9), AHC.

55. Report for Archives, Marillac Provincial House, 1967–68, ADOC; "A Tradition of Excellence."

56. "Moody Gift Puts Seton 'Over Top,'" AF Hospitals—Seton—H2770 (9), 1974, AHC; Sister Mary Rose to Doctors, July 17, 1964, ADOC.

57. "Seton Today," *Austin American-Statesman*, January 7, 1979. Elora Watt Smith was the first chair of the Seton Development Board.

58. "A Tradition of Excellence"; Sister Gertrude Levy and Christopher J. Attal, "The Story of Seton: The Growth of Seton from Infirmary to Network," 2002; and "The Acquisition of Holy Cross Hospital," both in Central File, ADOC.

59. "Hospital Growth," February 28, 1969, newspaper clipping, ADOC.

60. *Seton Medical Center Annual Report*, Fiscal Year 1987, ADOC.

61. Ibid.; Levy and Attal, "The Story of Seton."

62. Daughters of Charity Health Services of Austin, *Care for the Poor and Community Benefit, 1991 Annual Report*, CAT.

63. Levy and Attal, "The Story of Seton."

64. Earl Golz, "Barnett Deftly Leading Seton's Charge into Future," *Austin American-Statesman*, August 16, 1998; Dana Smith, "An Interview with Seton's Charles Barnett," September 29, 2007, http://www.senioradvocatenews.com/article. cfm?articleID=17026. Accessed November 20, 2009.

65. Andrew Park, "Seton Extending Health-Care Reach," *Austin American-Statesman*, October 6, 1998.

66. Ibid.

67. Ibid. See also *1991 Annual Report*.

68. Seton Family of Hospitals Community Report, Austin, Texas, 2008.

69. Monica Langley, "Money Order: Nuns' Zeal for Profits Shapes Hospital Chain, Wins Wall Street Fans," *Wall Street Journal*, January 7, 1998.

70. Editorial, "Catholic Health Care Poised between Mission and Money," *National Catholic Reporter*, http://www.natcath.com/NCR_Online/archives/012398/012398f. htm. Accessed November 3, 2009.

71. Langley, "Money Order."

72. *Annual Reports of Management*, 1935, 1937–1940, 1945, Administration folder, UPMC/Mercy Archives.

73. Report of Management for the Years 1947–1951 and Annual Staff Meeting Mercy Hospital, January 19, 1950, Medical Staff Annual Reports file, both in UPMC/Mercy Archives.

74. Sister M. Ferdinand Clark, "A Hospital for the Black Ghetto," *Hospital Progress*, February 1969, 49–51; Kathleen Washy, "Catholic Health Care and Urban Renewal: Pittsburgh, Pennsylvania's Mercy Hospital, 1953–1978" (paper presented at the American Catholic Historical Association meeting, Spring 2003, Scranton, Pa.).

75. Biographical Information, Sister Ferdinand Clark, UPMC/Mercy Archives. Sister Ferdinand attended Mt. Mercy College but there is no record of her receiving a degree.

76. Sister M. Cornelius Meerwald, *History of the Pittsburgh Mercy Hospital, 1847–1959* (Pittsburgh: Sisters of Mercy, 1959); Rosenfeld Study, 1962, UPMC/Mercy Archives.

77. Code of Regulations—Advisory Board, Minutes of the Advisory Board of Mercy Hospital; Rosenfeld Study, 1962; "Joint Meeting of the Board of Trustees and the Advisory Board of Mercy Hospital," September 19, 1963, Board of Trustees/Advisory Board Minutes file; *Mercy Bulletin*, May 1964, all in UPMC/Mercy Archives. See also *Pillar of Pittsburgh: The History of Mercy Hospital and the City It Serves* (Pittsburgh: Sisters of Mercy, n.d.), 186; Jeanette Rafferty, *Mercy Hospital, 1847–1972: An Historical Review* (Pittsburgh: Mercy Hospital, 1974); and Sister Jerome McHale, *On the Wing: The Story of the Pittsburgh Sisters of Mercy, 1843–1968* (New York: Seabury Press, 1980).

78. *Pillar of Pittsburgh*, 147; Hospital Planning Association of Allegheny County, Board of Directors Meeting, May 23, 1960, New Mercy Hospital File, UPMC/Mercy Archives. The HPA had.

79. Minutes, Hospital Planning Association, August 26, 1969; Memorandum from Sister M. Ferdinand to All Department Heads, April 22, 1971, HPA file; and "Mercy Hospital Progress Report to the Hospital Planning Association, November 1972, all in UPMC/Mercy Archives.

80. Information Summary for Meeting with Mr. Schaffer, February 3, 1971, Mercy Hospital of Pittsburgh file, UMPC/Mercy Archives; and *Pillar of Pittsburgh*.

81. Meerwald, *History of the Pittsburgh Mercy Hospital*; *Pillar of Pittsburgh*; History of the Department of Pastoral Care, 1974, Mission Services: Pastoral Care Histories file, UPMC/Mercy Archives.

82. Eastern Mercy Health System, April 1989 Organization Chart, 4/3 AR 1988–89 file; PMHS Chart, 4/3 AR 1990 file; and Pittsburgh Mercy Health System Organization Chart, February 21, 1994, all in UPMC/Mercy Archives. See also *Pittsburgh Catholic Special Supplement*, May 8, 1987, 2–3; Pittsburgh Mercy, A Heritage of Hope, http://www.pmhs.org/mcauleyministries/history.aspx. Accessed March 27, 2009.

83. James C. Robinson, "Entrepreneurial Challenges to Integrated Health Care," in *Policy Challenges in Modern Health Care*, ed. David Mechanic, Lynn B. Rogut, David C. Colby, and James R. Knickman (New Brunswick, N.J.: Rutgers University Press, 2005), 53–67.

84. Ik-Whan Kwon, Scott R. Safranski, David G. Martin, and William R. Walker, "Causes of Financial Difficulty in Catholic Hospitals," *Health Care Management*

Review 13, no. 1 (1988): 29–37. Pittsburgh Mercy Health System, Inc. Status Report, October 18, 1990; *1993 Annual Report,* April 21, 1994; and *Pittsburgh Mercy Health System Annual Report of the President/CEO,* 4/3 AR 1990, 1993 folders, all in UPMC/Mercy Archives.

85. Marc Hopkins, "Area Health Field Remains Chaotic," *Pittsburgh Business Times,* May 13, 1996.

86. Suzanne Elliott, "More Hospitals Talk of Getting Together," *Pittsburgh Tribune-Review,* May 3, 1996; Marc Hopkins, "UPMC Prepared to Spend $300 Million for Hospitals," *Pittsburgh Business Times,* March 18, 1996; William H. Maruca and Edward J. Kabala, "Healthcare Consolidation—Western Pennsylvania Style," *Hospital and Healthcare News,* June 1996, C-1.

87. Jane-Eleen Robinet, "Mercy, West Penn Form New Network," *Pittsburgh Business Times,* September 16–22, 1996; Pamela Gaynor, "Hospital Venture Fell Through on Merger," *Pittsburgh Post-Gazette,* August 13, 1997.

88. James C. Robinson discusses similar challenges to other hospitals in "Entrepreneurial Challenges."

89. Lawton R. Burns, John Cacciamani, James Clement, and Welman Aquino, "The Fall of the House of AHERF: The Allegheny Bankruptcy," *Health Affairs* 19, no. 1 (January–February 2000): 7–41; Pamela Gaynor, "AGH Pushes Back Deadline for Picking Merger Partner," *Pittsburgh Post-Gazette,* January 23, 1999.

90. Memorandum from Sister Joanne Marie Andiorio to Members, Board of Trustees, "Annual Report of the President/CEO," 4/3 AR 1997 file, UPMC/Mercy Archives; Gaynor, "AGH Pushes Back Deadline"; and Pamela Gaynor and Christopher Snowbeck, "One Bidder Still Interested in AGH," *Pittsburgh Post-Gazette,* February 6, 1999.

91. Luis Fabregas, "St. Francis Blocks Plan for Partnership with Mercy," *Tribune Review,* April 4, 2000; "Health Systems Talk Joint Venture," *Pittsburgh Tribune-Review,* August 8, 2001; Pamela Gaynor, "Hospital Merger Plan Collapses: St. Francis Options Few as Mercy Ends Talks," *Pittsburgh Post-Gazette,* January 31, 2002; Chuck Moody, "St. Francis Health System Sale Opens New Chapter of Health Care," *Pittsburgh Catholic,* August 23, 2002. These sources are also available in "Clippings Collection: Network Possibilities," UPMC/Mercy Archives.

92. Christopher Snowbeck and Joe Fahy, "Mercy Initiated Merger Talks with UPMC to Stay Open," *Pittsburgh Post-Gazette,* September 22, 2006; McCauley Ministries, History, http://www.pmhs.org/mcauley-ministries/history.aspx. Accessed March 27, 2009.

93. McCauley Ministries, History, http://www.pmhs.org/mcauley-ministries/history .aspx. Accessed March 27, 2009.

94. Peter J. Cunningham, Gloria J. Bazzoli, and Aaron Katz, "Caught in the Competitive Crossfire: Safety-Net Providers Balance Margin and Mission in a Profit-Driven Health Care Market," *Health Affairs*—Web Exclusive, August 12, 2008, w374–w382. See also Fitzhugh Mullan, "Still Closing the Gap," *Health Affairs* 28, no. 4 (July–August 2009): 1183–1188.

95. 1921 advertisement, Box HC 1.1, SMA.

96. Brief Dated History of Mercy Hospital Chicago, Mother Huberta McCarthy's Notes, Box HC 1.1, SMA; Joy Clough, *In Service to Chicago: The History of Mercy Hospital* (Chicago: Mercy Hospital and Medical Center, 1979).

97. Letter to Rev. T. H. Ahearn, November 16, 1932, Box HC 1.1, SMA; Clough, *In Service to Chicago*.

98. Mercy Free Dispensary, Sister M. Lorenzo to Mother Domitilla, March 12, 1954, Box HC 1.12, SMA; Brief Dated History of Mercy Hospital Chicago; Clough, *In Service to Chicago*.

99. Mother Mary Regina Cunningham, "Mercy Hospital," November 1958; "A Brief History of Mercy Hospital," for Cardinal Meyer, February 1959; and Letter to Cardinal Meyer, May 13, 1961, all in Box HC 1.12, #3, SMA.

100. "A Brief History"; History of Stritch School of Medicine, http://www.meddean .luc.edu/node/105. Accessed November 20, 2009. See also Clough, *In Service to Chicago*.

101. Clough, *In Service to Chicago*.

102. Massey and Denton, *American Apartheid*, 67–71; Clough, *In Service to Chicago*.

103. *1981 Annual Report* and *1985 Annual Report*, Mercy Hospital and Medical Center, MHA.

104. While Sister Sheila was health commissioner, the infant mortality rate for Chicago decreased from 17 per one thousand live births to 10.4.

105. Bruce Japsen, "Catholics Urge Hospitals to Stay Not-for-Profit," *Modern Healthcare* 30 (November 13, 1995), n.p.

106. Selected Works of Joseph Cardinal Bernardin, "A Sign of Hope: Pastoral Letter on Health Care," http://books.google.com/books?id=2aTqG1uajf0C&pg=PA81&lp g=PA81&dq=cardinal+bernardin+a+sign+of+hope&source=bl&ots=cK8CCcEPbI &sig=slPfEu-61zeK35ytpLv8cL7aT5M&hl=en&ei=arPyS9eeGMOclgfH4uiBDQ&s a=X&oi=book_result&ct=result&resnum=1&ved=0CBIQ6AEwAA#v=onepage&q =cardinal%20bernardin%20a%20sign%200f%20hope&f=false. Accessed May 17, 2009.

107. Peter J. W. Elstrom, "Hospital's Investment on Sick List," *Crain's Chicago Business*, July 22, 1991, 1; Della de Lafuente, "Cardinal's Rules Limit Hospitals' Plans to Merge," *Chicago Sun Times*, September 19, 1994; and Meera Somasundaram, "Hospital, Heal Thyself: New Team Aims to Revive Mercy's Finances," *Crain's Chicago Business*, April 19, 1999, 4, 53.

108. Mercy sources are silent as to what the "mistakes" were. This financial mismanagement was not typical of lay-religious administration of hospitals; most were effective.

109. Bruce Japsen, "Mercy's Losses Force Job Cuts," *Chicago Tribune*, April 27, 2000. Two lay executives held the chief management positions from 1994 to 1999. The consultants were Arthur Andersen and Wellspring Partners.

110. Sister Sheila Lyne, telephone interview by author, May 29, 2009.

111. Ibid.

112. Bruce Japsen, "Mercy Hospital Looks to End Independence," *Chicago Tribune*, October 24, 2002; Nancy Kennedy, "Sister Sheila Lyne Supports Staff with Spiritual Care Center," *Chicago Hospital News*, August 2004, 1; Bruce Japsen, "Mercy Counting Its Blessings," *Chicago Tribune*, August 11, 2008.

113. Lyne interview.

114. Ibid. "Lyne Shines on a Mission for Mercy," May 10, 2002, Box HC 1.27, #2, SMA; Bruce Japsen, "Mercy Hospital's For-Profit Shift Awaits Archdiocese's OK," *Chicago Tribune*, April 24, 2003; "Financial Upturn Gives Mercy Time to Freshen Up for Potential Suitors," *Chicago Tribune*, December 4, 2004.

115. Bruce Japsen, "Mercy Hospital Resumes Payment on Bonds," *Chicago Tribune*, March 25, 2004; Japsen, "Mercy Counting Its Blessings."

116. Statistics and Studies, http://www.aha.org/aha/resource-center/Statistics-and-Studies/fast-facts.html. Accessed July 17, 2009. Of the 4,897 U.S. community hospitals in 2007, 4,202 (86 percent) were members of a system or network.

117. Langley, "Money Order"; Lyne interview.

118. Robinson, "Entrepreneurial Challenges."

119. Ibid.; Risse, *Mending Bodies, Saving Souls.*

120. Sister Doris Gottemoeller, "Preserving Our Catholic Identity," *Health Progress* 80, no. 3 (May–June 1999), n.p. Article accessed May 15, 2009, at http://www.chausa.org/Pub/MainNav/News/HP/Archive/1999/05MayJune/Articles/Feature.

121. Robinson, "Entrepreneurial Challenges," 55.

122. Kenneth R. White, S. D. Roggenkamp, and A. J. LeBlanc, "Urban U.S. Hospitals and the Mission to Provide HIV-Related Services: Changes in Correlates," *Journal of Healthcare Management* 47, no. 1 (January–February 2002): 27–40; Kenneth R. White, Clarke E. Cochran, and Urvashi B. Patel, "Hospital Provision of End-of-Life Services: Who, What, and Where?" *Medical Care* 40, no. 1 (2002): 17–25.

Chapter 3 — Religion, Gender, and the Public Representation of Catholic Hospitals

1. Colleen McDannell, *Material Christianity: Religion and Popular Culture in America* (New Haven and London: Yale University Press, 1995), 1–2.

2. Barbra Mann Wall, *Unlikely Entrepreneurs: Catholic Sisters and the Hospital Marketplace, 1865–1925* (Columbus: Ohio State University Press, 2005); Clarke E. Cochran, "Another Identity Crisis: Catholic Hospitals Face Hard Choices," *Commonweal*, February 25, 2000, 12–15.

3. Samantha J. E. Riches and Sarah Salih, eds., *Gender and Holiness: Men, Women, and Saints in Late Medieval Europe* (London and New York: Routledge, 2002); Maxine Leeds Craig and Rita Liberti, " 'Cause that's what girls do': The Making of a Feminized Gym," *Gender and Society* 21, no. 5 (October 2007): 676–699; Cinzia Solari, "Professionals and Saints: How Immigrant Careworkers Negotiate Gender Identities at Work," *Gender and Society* 20, no. 3 (June 2006): 301–331.

4. Wall, *Unlikely Entrepreneurs.*

5. McDannell, *Material Christianity*, 142.

6. Richard P. McBrien, *Harper Collins Encyclopedia of Catholicism* (San Francisco: HarperCollins Publishers, 1995), 414; Ann Taves, *The Household of Faith: Roman Catholic Devotions in Mid-Nineteenth Century America* (Notre Dame, Ind.: University of Notre Dame Press, 1986), 30; James M. O'Toole, ed., *Habits of Devotion: Catholic Religious Practice in Twentieth-Century America* (Ithaca, N.Y.: Cornell University Press, 2004).

7. McDannell, *Material Christianity.*

8. Linda Fannin, "Seton's New Center Impressive Facility," *Austin American-Statesman*, May 11, 1975; "A Gift of Beauty," *Seton Today*, n.d. See also John O'Connell, "Volunteers Smooth Seton Hospital Transfer," *Austin American-Statesman*, March 24, 1975. Copies of these newspaper articles are located in AHC.

9. Roger Finke and Rodney Stark, *The Churching of America, 1776–1990: Winners and Losers in Our Religious Economy* (New Brunswick, N.J.: Rutgers University Press, 1992).

10. Paula Kane, "Marian Devotion since 1940: Continuity or Casualty?" In *Habits of Devotion*, ed. O'Toole, 89–129.

11. Jay P. Dolan, *The American Catholic Experience: A History from Colonial Times to the Present* (Notre Dame, Ind.: University of Notre Dame Press, 1992), 388; McDannell, *Material Christianity*, chapter 6.

12. Philip Gleason, *Keeping the Faith: American Catholicism Past and Present* (Notre Dame, Ind.: University of Notre Dame Press, 1987), 78 (quotation), 87–88. Dolan, *The American Catholic Experience*.

13. Sister Daniel Hannefin, *Daughters of the Church: A Popular History of the Daughters of Charity in the United States, 1809–1987* (New York: New City Press, 1989).

14. History, Carlow University, http://www.carlow.edu/about-carlow/history/index.html. Accessed May 18, 2009.

15. *Footnotes, Mercy Hospital and Medical Center, Chicago, Illinois*, Spring 1975, n.p., MHA.

16. *Pillar of Pittsburgh: The History of Mercy Hospital and the City It Serves* (Pittsburgh: Sisters of Mercy, n.d.); Porte Cochere brochure, UPMC/Mercy Archives.

17. C. A. Hangartner, "Implications for Nursing Education from Vatican II," *Hospital Progress* 47 (October 1966): 63–66, 78.

18. *63rd Annual Report*, 1928; and *74th Annual Report*, 1939, ABA.

19. Excerpts from article in *Chicago Tribune*, August 25, 1880, ABA.; Hospital Statistics, 1942, ABA.

20. Lawrence Davidson, *The Alexian Brothers of Chicago: An Evolutionary Look at the Monastery and Modern Health Care* (New York: Vantage Press, 1990), 72.

21. *86th Annual Report*, 1951, 7, ABA.

22. Christopher J. Kauffman, *Ministry and Meaning: A Religious History of Catholic Health Care in the United States* (New York: Crossroad, 1995).

23. *75th Annual Report*, 1940; *85th Annual Report*, 1950, ABA.

24. *85th Annual Report*, 9, ABA.

25. *The Golden Sheaf, Providence Hospital, 1877–1927*, 39, PSMC Archives.

26. Alphonse Schwitalla, "Present Problems of Catholic Schools of Nursing and Hospitals," *Hospital Progress* 18 (September 1938): 301.

27. Susan Reverby, *Ordered to Care: The Dilemma of American Nursing, 1850–1945* (New York: Cambridge University Press, 1987); Patricia D'Antonio, *American Nursing: A History of Knowledge, Authority, and the Meaning of Work* (Baltimore: Johns Hopkins University Press, 2010).

28. Chad E. O'Lynn and Russell E. Tranbarger, eds., *Men in Nursing: History, Challenges, and Opportunities* (New York: Springer, 2007).

29. Mary Roberts, *American Nursing: History and Interpretation* (New York: Macmillan, 1955); M. Gijswijt-Hofstra, H. Oosterhuis, J. Vijselaar, and H. Freeman, eds., *Psychiatric Cultures Compared: Psychiatry and Mental Health Care in the Twentieth Century* (Amsterdam: Amsterdam University Press, 2005).

30. *Diaconian* (yearbook), 1966, 59, ABA.

31. Riches and Salih, *Gender and Holiness*.

32. *75th Annual Report*; *Hospital Statistics*, 1942; *85th Annual Report*, all in ABA.

33. Julia T. Wood, *Who Cares? Women, Care, and Culture* (Carbondale: Southern Illinois University Press, 1994); C. D. McGraw, "'Every nurse is not a sister': Sex, Work and the Invention of the Spanish American War Nurse" (PhD diss., University of Connecticut, 2005).

34. Carol Gilligan, *In a Different Voice: Psychological Theory and Women's Development* (Cambridge, Mass.: Harvard University Press, 1982); Nel Noddings, *Caring—A Feminine Approach to Ethics and Moral Education* (Berkeley: University of California Press, 1984); Wood, *Who Cares?* 20.

35. Judith Lorber and Jeffrey C. Alexander, *Breaking the Bowls: Degendering and Feminist Change* (New York: Norton, 2005).

36. Kauffman, *Ministry and Meaning.*

37. *61st Annual Report*, 1926; *63rd Annual Report*; *74th Annual Report*, all in ABA.

38. School of Nursing Monthly Meetings, 1925; *Diary, Alexian Brothers School of Nursing*; *74th Annual Report*; *91st Annual Report*, 1956, all in ABA. The *Diary* was compiled by Brother Sebastian Brogan John Blackledge.

39. Davidson, *The Alexian Brothers of Chicago.*

40. *Diary*, 1929.

41. Davidson, *The Alexian Brothers of Chicago.*

42. *Diary*, 1929.

43. *Diary*, June 7, 1938; *Diaconian*, 1954, 1969; "Catholic Health Association Annual Report, 1985–1986," copy in ABA.

44. Davidson, *The Alexian Brothers of Chicago.* Minutes of the General Chapter Meeting, 1932; and Ignatius Wiegers, "History of the Aachen Alexian Brothers, Aachen, Germany" (1995), both in ABA.

45. *Diary*, June 7, 1938, and January 12, 1939; Davidson, *The Alexian Brothers of Chicago.*

46. *74th Annual Report; Diary*, entry for September 8, 1939, both in ABA.

47. "Two Year's Service for the Sick at Alexian in I-W, Alexian Brother's I-W Unit," n.d., probably 1943, microfilm copy, ABA.

48. R. A. Lion and B. T. Bell, "Three Years of CPS Unit #26 (March 1, 1945)," ABA.

49. "Two Year's Service for the Sick," ABA.

50. *Diary*, February 14, 1947; *85th Annual Report*, ABA.

51. "Now Men Assert Rights," Newspaper Clippings file, n.d., ABA.

52. Christine L. Williams, *Gender Differences at Work: Women and Men in Non-Traditional Occupations* (Berkeley: University of California Press, 1989); Christine L. Williams, ed., *Doing "Women's Work": Men in Nontraditional Occupations* (Newbury Park, Calif.: Sage Publications, 1993); Christine L. Williams, *Still a Man's World: Men Who Do "Women's" Work* (Berkeley: University of California Press, 1995); Robin Leidner, *Fast Food, Fast Talk: Service Work and the Routinization of Everyday Life* (Berkeley: University of California Press, 1993).

53. Solari, "Professionals and Saints," 311.

54. *85th Annual Report*, ABA.

55. T. J. Kaveny, "Valedictory Address: Guidebook for a Wartime Graduate," *The Alexian*, July 1942, 4, 5, ABA.

56. Mary Sarnecky, *A History of the US Army Nurse Corps* (Philadelphia: University of Pennsylvania Press, 1999).

57. "Memorable Events," *Diaconian*, 1952, 26, ABA.

58. M. F. Ferguson, *Diaconian*, 1955, 21, ABA.

59. Davidson, *The Alexian Brothers of Chicago.*

60. Williams, *Gender Differences, Doing Women's Work*, and *Still a Man's World.*

61. B. J. Welker, "A Study of Employer Preferences and Characteristics of the Graduates of the Alexian Brothers Hospital School of Nursing," *Diaconian*, 1969, 67, ABA.

62. *Diaconian*, 1948; 1954; 1969, 59.

63. *Diaconian*, 1969, 59.

64. Solari, "Professionals and Saints."

65. Francine M. Deutsch, "Undoing Gender," *Gender and Society* 21 (2007): 106–127.

66. Rosemary Stevens, *In Sickness and in Wealth: American Hospitals in the Twentieth Century* (Baltimore: Johns Hopkins University Press, 1989; repr. 1999), 14.

Chapter 4 — Regardless of Color, Race, Creed, or Financial Status

1. "There Is a Christian Way to Run a Hospital," *New World*, 1955, Newspaper Clippings file, ABA.

2. Barbra Mann Wall, *Unlikely Entrepreneurs: Catholic Sisters and the Hospital Marketplace, 1865–1925* (Columbus: Ohio State University Press, 2005).

3. *Pub. L. 88–352, title VI, Sec. 601, July 2, 1964, 78 Stat. 252*, http://www.usdoj.gov/crt/cor/coord/titlevistat.htm. Accessed April 27, 2008.

4. Quintard Taylor, *The Forging of a Black Community: Seattle's Central District from 1870 through the Civil Rights Era* (Seattle: University of Washington Press, 1994); and James N. Gregory, "Seattle Civil Rights and Labor History Project," http://depts.washington.edu/civilr/. Accessed February 8, 2009.

5. As new black residents competed with Catholics for jobs and housing, racial hostilities erupted in violence. See John T. McGreevy, *Parish Boundaries: The Catholic Encounter with Race in the Twentieth-Century Urban North* (Chicago: University of Chicago Press, 1996); Thomas J. Sugrue, *Sweet Land of Liberty: The Forgotten Struggle for Civil Rights in the North* (New York: Random House, 2008).

6. Douglas S. Massey and Nancy A. Denton, *American Apartheid: Segregation and the Making of the Underclass* (Cambridge, Mass.: Harvard University Press, 1993).

7. Vanessa N. Gamble, *Making a Place for Ourselves: The Black Hospital Movement, 1920–1945* (New York: Oxford University Press, 1995); Darlene Clark Hine, *Black Women in White: Racial Conflict and Cooperation in the Nursing Profession, 1890–1950* (Bloomington: Indiana University Press, 1989); Steven Avella, *This Confident Church: Catholic Leadership and Life in Chicago, 1940–1965* (Notre Dame, Ind.: University of Notre Dame Press, 1992); "Chicago Friendship House Report on Discrimination of Catholic Hospitals," September 1955, Friendship House Papers, Box 15, Undated Items folder, CHM.

8. Eugene H. Bradley, "Health, Hospitals, and the Negro," *Modern Hospital* 65, no. 2 (August 1945): 43–44.

9. The U.S. Supreme Court struck down the "separate but equal" clause of the Hill-Burton Act in 1963. See "The Hill-Burton Act and Civil Rights: Expanding Hospital Care for Black Southerners, 1939–1960," *Journal of Southern History*, November 1, 2006, http://goliath.ecnext.com/coms2/gi_0199–6005519/The-Hill_Burton_Act-and.html. Accessed October 23, 2009; Max Seham, "Discrimination against Negroes in Hospitals," *New England Journal of Medicine* 271, no. 18 (1964): 940–943; E. H. Beardsley, "Good-Bye to Jim Crow: The Desegregation of Southern Hospitals, 1945–1970," *Bulletin of the History of Medicine* 60 (1986): 367–386.

10. Paul B. Cornely, "Trends in Racial Integration in Hospitals in the United States," *Journal of the National Medical Association* 49, no. 1 (January 1957): 8–10.

11. U.S. Department of Health, Education, and Welfare, *Vital Statistics of the United States*, 1960, vol. 2, *Mortality*, Part A (Washington, D.C.: Public Health Service, 1963), 1–6, 2–6, tables 1-E, 3-A, 3-C, 3-E.

12. "Non-Segregation Works at St. Vincent's, Kansas City," *Hospital Progress* 34 (November 1953): 47–49; Suzy Farren, *A Call to Care: The Women Who Built Catholic Healthcare in America* (St. Louis: Catholic Health Association of the United States, 1996); John M. Vietoris, " 'A Golden Opportunity for Reaping a Harvest of Souls': A History of the Ministry to African American Catholics in Milwaukee, 1908–1963" (PhD diss., Marquette University, March 2009). Suellen Hoy has shown how some women's teaching congregations were successful in working with blacks in mid-twentieth-century Chicago, including the Sisters of the Good Shepherd, who opted to stay in the inner city when other whites left. See Suellen Hoy, *Good Hearts: Catholic Sisters in Chicago's Past* (Urbana: University of Illinois Press, 2006).

13. A. R. Hirsch, *Making the Second Ghetto: Race and Housing in Chicago, 1940–1960* (Chicago: University of Chicago Press, 1998); Hine, *Black Women in White*, 31.

14. "Protest Atrocities in Local Hospitals," *Chicago Daily Defender*, July 24, 1926; "Would Stop Segregation in Hospitals," *Chicago Defender*, May 7, 1927; Vanessa Northington Gamble, "The Provident Hospital Project: An Experiment in Race Relations and Medical Education," *Bulletin of the History of Medicine* 65 (1991): 457–475.

15. McGreevy, *Parish Boundaries*; Avella, *This Confident Church*.

16. Mrs. Maude Johnston to Most Reverend Samuel A. Stritch, March 23, 1944, Friendship House Papers, Box 1, Jan–May 1944 folder, CHM.

17. "Board of Trustees Meeting," The Mercy and Mercy Orphan Asylum, Chicago, Illinois, June 7, 1949, Box HC 1.3, #12, ASM.

18. Avella, *This Confident Church*.

19. A. M. Mercer, Inaugural Address, January 1950, Chancery Correspondence, 1/1/195–12/31/195, Box Mc-M, Archives of the Archdiocese of Chicago, Chicago, Ill.

20. *1952 Annual Report*, Mercy Hospital; Mercy Hospital Newsletter, August 1958, both in MHA.

21. Archbishop Stritch to Rev. Daniel Cantwell, October 26, 1955, CHM; His Eminence Samuel Cardinal Stritch, "Interracial Justice in Hospitals," *Interracial Review*, November 1955, n.p, Cantwell Papers, Box 9, folder 9–3, CHM.

22. Report from Catholic Interracial Council, probably 1955, Friendship House Papers, Box 15, Undated Items folder, CHM.

23. Catholic Interracial Council report, August 28, 1956, CIC Collection, Box 13, August 1956 folder, CHM [hereafter CIC report, 1956].

24. Anthony Vader, "Racial Segregation within Catholic Institutions in Chicago: A Study in Behavior and Attitudes" (MA thesis, University of Chicago, School of Sociology, 1962). See also CIC report, 1956.

25. Amy L. Koehlinger, *The New Nuns: Racial Justice and Religious Reform in the 1960s* (Cambridge, Mass.: Harvard University Press, 2007), 168.

26. CIC report, 1956.

27. Ibid.

28. Ibid.

29. Vader, "Racial Segregation within Catholic Institutions."

30. "Acts of the General Chapter, 1920 and 1926, Pro-1, Box 4, folder 3, ABA. The archives are silent as to why the brothers made this decision.

31. Council Minutes, February 1, 1953, ABA; photographs of the 1954 diploma nursing school first-year class, MHA; *Chronicles*, 1952–1985, (56), PSMC, SPA. A 1950

agreement gave administration to Seattle University with clinical practice at Providence Hospital, making it the Providence Unit.

32. "Local Hospital Shifts to Segregation," *Chicago Daily Defender*, n.d., Newspaper Clippings file, ABA.

33. Quoted in Lawrence Davidson, *The Alexian Brothers of Chicago: An Evolutionary Look at the Monastery and Modern Health Care* (New York: Vantage Press, 1990), 169.

34. Report to the Catholic Interracial Council, Tuesday, August 28, 1956, folder labeled August 1956, CIC Papers, CHM.

35. Sugrue, *Sweet Land of Liberty*.

36. U.S. Conference of Catholic Bishops, "Discrimination and the Christian Conscience," 1958. See *Bryan N. Massingale, Racial Justice and the Catholic Church* (Maryknoll, N.Y.: Orbis Books, 2010).

37. "Chicago's Hospital Bias," *Chicago Daily Defender*, March 24, 1958; "Hospitals Snub Negro Medics," *Chicago Defender*, April 25, 1959.

38. Joy Clough, *In Service to Chicago: The History of Mercy Hospital* (Chicago: Mercy Hospital and Medical Center, 1979). Available sources do not reveal the outcome of the lawsuit.

39. Rosemary Stevens, *In Sickness and in Wealth: American Hospitals in the Twentieth Century* (Baltimore: Johns Hopkins University Press, 1989; repr. 1999), 315.

40. McGreevy, *Parish Boundaries*.

41. Andrew M. Greeley, "The Catholic Suburbanite," *The Sign* 37 (February 1958): 30; Donald R. Campion and Dennis Clark, "So You're Moving to Suburbia," *America*, April 21, 1956, 80–82.

42. Edward V. Ellis, "Changing Neighborhoods: The Challenge to Stay," *Hospital Progress*, January 1970, 43.

43. Massey and Denton, *American Apartheid*, 67–71.

44. Brother Flavian to Brother Provincial, February 27, 1961, Planning Committee Report, ABA.

45. Donald Dewey, *Where the Doctors Have Gone* (Chicago: Chicago Regional Hospital Study, Illinois Regional Medical Program, 1973).

46. Bruce Japsen, "Rankings Shed Light on Hospitals," *Chicago Tribune*, October 8, 1998; Bruce Japsen, "Hospitals Find Rankings a Pain," *Chicago Tribune*, October 14, 1998.

47. Clough, *In Service to Chicago*.

48. "The Quality of Mercy Not Strained at Hospital," *Chicago Daily News*, February 3, 1948; Admission Policy (from Admitting Office Manual), attached to letter from Sister Mary Venarda to Mr. Leo Tierney, April 13, 1961; Sister Mary Venarda to Mother Mary Huberta, April 22, 1961, both in ASM.

49. Seattle Civil Rights and Labor History Project, Segregated Seattle, http://depts .washington.edu/civilr/segregated.htm. Accessed February 27, 2009.

50. See, for example, *Chronicles*, 1902, 1905, (56), PSMC Collection, SPA.

51. "The Golden Sheath, Providence Hospital, 1877–1927," (56), PSMC Collection—History, SPA.

52. Ibid.

53. "Miss Uno Harbors No Ill-Feelings," *Japanese-American Courier*, August 25, 1928. Copy located in (1257) RPP, Box 8, Special Series, Institutions. See also Taylor, *The Forging of a Black Community*.

54. *Chronicles*, 1930, (56), PSMC Collection, SPA.

55. Stub Nelson, "Anti-Jap Move by Farmers Gains Force," *Seattle Star*, December 14, 1944. Reprinted in Jennifer Speidel, "After Internment: Seattle's Debate over Japanese Americans' Right to Return Home," http://depts.washington.edu/civilr/after_internment.htm. Accessed June 22, 2008.

56. *Chronicles*, March 2 and May 1, 1942, (56), PSMC Collection, SPA.

57. "The Problem of Student Nurses of Japanese Ancestry," *American Journal of Nursing* 43 (October 1943): 895; "Japanese-American Students," *American Journal of Nursing* 44 (1944): 72; "Students of Japanese Ancestry," *American Journal of Nursing* 46 (July 1946): 495.

58. *Chronicles*, March 13, 1945, Personnel/Employees, (61) St. Mary Hospital, Astoria, Oregon, Collection, SPA. See also "Japanese Back Home," *Astoria Evening Budget*, March 23, 1945. Microfilm copy from Astoria Public Library, Astoria, Ore., SPA.

59. Taylor, *The Forging of a Black Community*.

60. Ibid. See also National Association for the Advancement of Colored People (NAACP)—Seattle Branch, http://depts.washington.edu/civilr/organizations.htm#naacp. Accessed February 28, 2009.

61. Christian Friends for Racial Equality to Mr. G. M. Greenwood, March 19, 1945. National Association for the Advancement of Colored People (NAACP)—Seattle Branch, http://depts.washington.edu/civilr/organizations.htm#naacp. Accessed February 28, 2009; and *Chronicles*, 1952–1985, (56), PSMC Collection, SPA.

62. "Analysis of Hospital Service for the Year Ending December 31, 1955," Annual Report 1955, (56), PSMC, Box 29, Reports, Annual Medical Reports, SPA.

63. Maureen Sullivan, *The Road to Vatican II: Key Changes in Theology* (New York: Paulist Press; 2007), 14.

64. "Civil Rights Mass, March 2, 1964"; "Carl Rogers Workshop," August 23, 1967; "Chinese New Year," February 16, 1969, all in *Chronicles*, 1952–1985, (56), PSMC Collection SPA.

65. Taylor, *The Forging of a Black Community, 193*.

66. "Guards on Duty," March 31, 1970, *Chronicles*, 1952–1985, (56), PSMC Collection, SPA. See also Taylor, *The Forging of a Black Community*.

67. "Sisters Study Discrimination in Hospitals," November 30, 1972, news release from Bill Tobin, Director of Public Relations, Sisters of Providence Sacred Heart Province, (56), PSMC Collection, Box 32, Reports, SPA.

68. Massey and Denton, *American Apartheid*, 66.

69. Earl Belle Smith, "Medical Care and the Negro," *Journal of the National Medical Association* 54, no. 3 (1962): 393–395. Dr. Earl Belle Smith was president of the Interracial Council and chair of the Committee on Discrimination in Medicine of the National Catholic Conference for Interracial Justice.

70. Sister M. Ferdinand Clark, "A Hospital for the Black Ghetto," *Hospital Progress*, February 1969, 49; Kathleen Washy, "Catholic Health Care and Urban Renewal: Pittsburgh, Pennsylvania's Mercy Hospital, 1953–1978" (paper presented at the American Catholic Historical Association meeting, Spring 2003, Scranton, Pa.); *Pillar of Pittsburgh: The History of Mercy Hospital and the City It Serves* (Pittsburgh: Sisters of Mercy, n.d.). It is not known if blacks favored another plan.

71. Dorothy Anderson, "'Awful Set Up,' Patients Charge," *Pittsburgh Courier*, July 6, 1946; "Coal Company Studies Mercy Hospital Bias" and "Sister Mary Has No Comment for Courier," *Pittsburgh Courier*, July 13, 1946.

72. George E. Barbour, "Many Better-Than-Average Jobs Now Held by Negroes, Courier Survey Shows," *Pittsburgh Courier*, January 9, 1960; Thomas A. Hennessy, "Urban League Hits Doctor 'Inequality,'" *Pittsburgh Post-Gazette* [1963], "Clippings Collection: Network Possibilities," UPMC/Mercy Archives.

73. Sister Ferdinand, "A Hospital for the Black Ghetto"; Sister Ferdinand Clark to Neighborhood Committee Member, November 8, 1976; Sara Stanley to Sister Ferdinand Clark, Mailgram, November 15, 1976; Minutes of Neighborhood Committee on Health Care, November 18 and 22, 1976, all in Neighborhood Committee Health Care File, UPMC/Mercy Archives.

74. Sister Mary Ferdinand Clark, "Adequate Health Care: One Step toward Social Justice," *Hospital Progress*, October 1978, n.p.

75. Ibid.; Sister Ferdinand, "A Hospital for the Black Ghetto"; "Hospital Names 2 Negroes to Staff," *Pittsburgh Courier*, September 14, 1968; George Thomas, "Mercy Hospital Promises Outpatients 'New Deal,'" *Pittsburgh Press*, August 28, 1968; document entitled "Information from Mercy Hospital, October 23, 1968"; "Mercy Health Center Total Patient Visits," RG8—Planning, UPMC/Mercy Hospital Archives.

76. Clark, "Adequate Health Care"; "Annual Report of the Administrator for the Year 1969," Administration Annual Reports, 1960–1969, UPMC/Mercy Archives.

77. Gamble, *Making a Place for Ourselves*; "Black Hospital Movement in Alabama," *Encyclopedia of Alabama*, http://www.encylopediaofalabama.org/face/Article.jsp?id=h-2410. Accessed October 23, 2009.

78. Sisters of St. Joseph Who Served at Good Samaritan Hospital, Selma, Alabama, Selma Collection G13–1–4, Folder 1, ASSJR.

79. "The Sisters of St. Joseph: 50 Years on Your Missions," *Edmundite Missions*, March 1990, ASSJR; Sisters of St. Joseph Who Served at Good Samaritan Hospital.

80. "The Sisters of St. Joseph: 50 Years on Your Missions."

81. Father Casey to Mother Rose Miriam, April 6, 1944, Selma Collection, G13–1–1, Folder 8, ASSJR.

82. Good Samaritan Hospital and School of Nursing, Selma Collection, G13–1–1, Folder 9D, ASSJR.

83. Hine, *Black Women in White*.

84. Casey to Mother Rose Miriam.

85. A. Fitts, "Good Samaritan Hospital," *Impact!* 1980, 1 (newsletter).

86. Typed letter to Monsignor Randall, June 1, 1950, Selma Collection, G13–1–4, Folder 6, ASSJR.

87. Ibid.

88. Robert J. Norrell, *Up from History: The Life of Booker T. Washington* (Cambridge, Mass.: Harvard University Press, 2008).

89. Good Samaritan School of Practical Nursing brochure, Selma Collection, G13–1–1, Folder 9A, ASSJR.

90. J. Wright, news release, n.d., Folder 9B, ASSJR.

91. Good Samaritan School of Practical Nursing brochure.

92. Ibid.; "Good Samaritan Began Alabama's First School of Practical Nursing," *Your Edmundite Missions Newsletter*, 1966, 5, Selma Collection, G13–1–1, Folder 9E, ASSJR.

93. A. Fitts, "Graduates Pay Tribute to 'Good Sam's' School of Nursing," n.d. (probably 1981), Selma Collection, G13–1–1, ASSJR.

94. Gamble, *Making a Place for Ourselves.*

95. J. N. Couture, "Twelve Years in the Southern Missions, 1949," Selma Collection, Folder 8, G13–1–1, ASSJR.

96. J. G. Brinckman, "More Than a Good Samaritan," *Colored Harvest,* May 1958, 12–14, Folder 9E; Good Samaritan Hospital and School of Nursing, Folder 9D; "Analysis of Hospital Service," January 1–December 31, 1959, Folder 9F, all in Good Samaritan Hospital, Inc., Selma Collection, G13–1–1, ASSJR. See also Sisters of St. Joseph Rochester, "Sister Ensured Good Samaritan's Nurses Were Well Trained," *Bridge* 33 (Summer 2000): 4.

97. "5-year Comparison of Patient Care," *Good Samaritan Hospital Newsletter,* 1964, ASSJR.

98. Sister Mary Paul to My Dear Sisters and Friends, Selma Series, Box G-13-1-2, Folder 14, ASSJR; Gregory Nelson Hite, "The Hottest Places in Hell: The Catholic Church, the Alabama Voting Rights Campaign and Selma, Alabama, 1937–1965" (PhD diss., University of Virginia, 2002); C. A. Jamison, "A Woman of Good Will to Leave Canandaigua," *Daily Messenger,* June 8, 1988.

99. Sisters Mary Paul Geck, Barbara Lum, Josepha Twomey, and Catherine Teresa Martin, taped interview by author, April 11, 2008, Rochester, N.Y. There was not a Catholic hospital in Selma for whites only.

100. Koehlinger, *The New Nuns.*

101. *Chronicles of St. Elizabeth's Convent,* Selma Collection, G13–1–4, Folder 6, ASSJR.

102. Koehlinger, *The New Nuns.*

103. Geck, Lum, Twomey, and Martin interview; Sister Eleanor [Sister Barbara Lum] to Mom and Dad, May 19, September 18, October 20, October 29, 1963, and July 14, 1964, Selma Collection, G13–1–4, Folder 10, ASSJR.

104. Sister Mary Paul to My Dear Sisters and Friends.

105. Sister Eleanor to Mom and Dad, May 19, 1963.

106. Geck, Lum, Twomey, and Martin interview.

107. Ibid.

108. Sister Eleanor to Mom and Dad.

109. Geck, Lum, Twomey, and Martin interview; *Sisters in Selma: Bearing Witness for Change,* DVD, PBS Television documentary by Catholic News Service/U.S. Conference of Catholic Bishops, 2007, aired as part of PBS's Black History Month.

110. Geck, Lum, Twomey, and Martin interview; J. Cogley, "The Clergy Heeds a New Call," *New York Times Magazine,* May 2, 1965, 54.

111. Geck, Lum, Twomey, and Martin interview.

112. Ibid.; Sister M. Liguori, "In Retrospect," June 4, 1966, n.p., Selma Collection, G13–1–1, Folder 8A, ASSJR.

113. Geck, Lum, Twomey, and Martin interview; "Sister Still Remembers Smell," *Bridge* 33 (2000): 4.; Liguori, "In Retrospect."

114. Ibid.

115. *Sisters in Selma.*

116. Geck, Lum, Twomey, and Martin interview.

117. Liguori, "In Retrospect."

118. Geck, Lum, Twomey, and Martin interview. See also "Alabama Bishop Attacks Marches by Priests, Nuns," *New York Herald Tribune,* March 19, 1965.

119. Cogley, "The Clergy Heeds a New Call," 54.

120. *Sisters in Selma*; Ursula Stepsis and Dolores Liptak, eds., *Pioneer Healers: The History of Women Religious in American Health Care* (New York: Crossroad, 1989), 209–211.

121. Sister Margaret Adelaide to Sister Alma Joseph, February 18, 1966, Selma collection, G13–1–1, Folder 9B, ASSJR. See also *Good News!* June 9, 1966, Selma Collection, G13–1–1, Folder 9B, ASSJR.

122. "Administrator's Report, Good Samaritan Hospital," 1971, Selma Collection, G13–1–1, Folder 9C, ASSJR.

123. "Publicity Release Given to the Advisory Board, Medical Staff of Good Samaritan Hospital in Selma; Later, to Newspapers," Selma Collection, G13–1–1, Folder 9B, ASSJR.

124. Annual Board of Trustees Meeting, Good Samaritan Hospital, Inc., November 20, 1970, Selma Collection, G13–1–1, Folder 9C; Meeting of the General Council, December 21, 1971; Mother Agnes Cecelia to Rev. Paul Marin, January 4, 1972, Selma Collection, G13–1–1, Folder 9B, all in ASSJR.

125. "Good Samaritan Hospital Faces a Financial Crisis," *Catholic Week*, October 30, 1981.

126. "Today in Alabama," *Bridge* 3 (1990): n.p.; J. Martin, "Good Samaritan Closes," *Selma Times Journal*, June 19, 1983; J. Walburn, "Hospital Matched Its Name for 61 Years," *Selma Times Journal*, June 19, 1983, all in ASSJR.

127. "The Sisters of St. Joseph: 50 Years on Your Missions"; Geck, Lum, Twomey, and Martin interview.

128. Koehlinger, *The New Nuns*.

129. Hoy, *Good Hearts*, 123.

130. Gamble, *Making a Place for Ourselves*.

131. Stepsis and Liptak, *Pioneer Healers*.

Chapter 5 — Catholic Hospitals and the Federal Government

1. U.S. Conference of Catholic Bishops, "Faithful Reform in Health Care," 1981, http://www.faithfulreform.org/index.php/Theology-and-Policy/United States Conference of Catholic Bishops United. Accessed January 30, 2009.

2. Jay P. Dolan, *The American Catholic Experience: A History of Colonial Times to the Present* (Notre Dame, Ind.: University of Notre Dame Press, 1992).

3. Michael V. Angrosino, "The Catholic Church and U.S. Health Care Reform," *Medical Anthropology Quarterly* 10, no. 1 (1996): 3–19.

4. Charles Morris, *American Catholic: The Saints and Sinners Who Built America's Most Powerful Church* (New York: Vintage Books, 1997); Garry Wills, *Head and Heart: A History of Christianity in America* (New York: Penguin Books, 2007).

5. See, for example, Alphonse Schwitalla, "The Catholic Hospital Association," *Hospital Progress*, March 1946, 75.

6. Rosemary Stevens, *In Sickness and in Wealth: American Hospitals in the Twentieth Century* (Baltimore: Johns Hopkins University Press, 1989; repr. 1999).

7. Christopher Kauffman, *Ministry and Meaning: A Religious History of Catholic Health Care in the United States* (New York: Crossroad, 1995).

8. Biographical sheet, Sister John Gabriel, RN, AB (1257), RPP, Box 2, Biography, Biographical Notes. Her books include *Through the Patient's Eyes: Hospitals, Doctors, Nurses* (Philadelphia: J. B. Lippincott, 1935); *Professional Problems: A Text-book for Nurses* (Philadelphia: W. B. Saunders, 1932); *Principles of Teaching in Schools*

of Nursing (New York: Macmillan, 1928); *Practical Methods of Study: A Textbook for Student Nurses* (New York: Macmillan, 1930); and *Teachers' Work Organization Book* (Philadelphia: W. B. Saunders, 1931).

9. Stevens, *In Sickness and in Wealth*; biographical sheet, Sister John Gabriel. See also Sister Miriam Teresa, SP, to Sister Joan Frances, SP, July 28, 1958, RPP, Box 2, Biography, Miscellaneous Correspondence, SPA.

10. Alphonse Schwitalla, "Last Year's and Next Year's Work," *Hospital Progress*, June 1931, 236–237; Robert J. Shanahan, *The History of the Catholic Hospital Association, 1915–1965: Fifty Years of Progress* (St. Louis: Catholic Hospital Association, 1965).

11. Sister M. Robert, "Hospital Economics: Depression and Its Effect on the Hospital," *Hospital Progress*, August 1931, 320.

12. "Hospital Service in the United States: Twelfth Annual Presentation of Hospital Data by the Council on Medical Education and Hospitals of the American Medical Association," *JAMA* 100, no. 12 (1933): 887. The Council on Medical Education and Hospitals asserted in 1933 that the country was "over hospitalized."

13. Phil Rheinecker, "Crisis and Reconstruction: The Depression and Catholic Hospitals," in *A Commitment to Healthcare: Celebrating 75 Years of the Catholic Health Association of the United States*, ed. Christopher Kauffman (St. Louis: Catholic Health Association of the United States, 1990), 29–30.

14. American Hospital Association, "President's Address," *Transactions of the American Hospital Association* (1932): 147.

15. Ibid.; Kauffman, *A Commitment to Healthcare*, 32.

16. Stevens, *In Sickness and in Wealth*, 163.

17. Shanahan, *The History of the Catholic Hospital Association*. The National Catholic Welfare Conference, developed in 1919, was the precursor to the National Conference of Catholic Bishops, organized in 1966.

18. Stevens, *In Sickness and in Wealth*.

19. "U.S. Aid in Care of Indigents Asked by Catholic Group," *Hospital Management* 38, no. 1 (July 1934): 43.

20. Stevens, *In Sickness and in Wealth*.

21. The Catholic Hospital Association, "Resolution XXXIX, the CHA Convention, the Care of the Indigent," *Hospital Progress*, July 1933, 287.

22. "U.S. Aid in Care of Indigents," 34. See also Shanahan, *The History of the Catholic Hospital Association*, 119, 121; Kauffman, *A Commitment to Healthcare*, 34.

23. Sister John Gabriel, "The Role of the Hospitals in the Recovery Program," *Hospital Management* 37 (May 1934): 36. Sister John Gabriel served as an advisory editorial staff member for this journal. See also Stevens, *In Sickness and in Wealth*.

24. Sister John Gabriel, "The Role of the Hospitals," 37.

25. Ibid., 38.

26. "U.S. Aid in Care of Indigents"; Shanahan, *The History of the Catholic Hospital Association*.

27. Shanahan, *The History of the Catholic Hospital Association*, 118–121; Copy of "Taxing Provision of the Social Security Act," extracted from December *Hospitals* (approx. 1935), (1257) RPP, Box 8, Legislation, Publications, Reports, and Notes, SPA. The committee said it wanted the exemption to have further opportunity to study any benefits to be gained by the taxes. See also "The Week's Trend in Hospital Legislation," March 4, 1935, (1257) RPP, Box 3, Correspondence, Speeches, and Writings, Nursing Education, SPA. See also Stevens, *In Sickness and in Wealth*.

28. "Sister John Gabriel: A Leader in a Time of Change," *Sisters of Providence Caritas* 14, no. 1 (January 1976): 1, Box 8, Legislation, Publications, Reports, and Notes, SPA.

29. Sister John Gabriel. "A Letter Which Helped to Kill Dangerous Bill," n.d., (1257) RPP, Box 8, Legislation, Correspondence, SPA.

30. James M. Geraghty to Sister John [of the Cross], July 7, 1939, (1257) RPP, Box 2, Biography, Miscellaneous Correspondence, SPA. Sister John Gabriel, rather than "taking" a male name, was assigned the religious name by her superior. Sometimes sisters suggested options for their religious names, which might include a combination of their father's and mother's names or names of male or female saints.

31. Carol K. Coburn and Martha Smith, *Spirited Lives: How Nuns Shaped Catholic Culture and American Life, 1836–1920* (Chapel Hill: University of North Carolina Press, 1999), 82–83.

32. Stevens, *In Sickness and in Wealth.*

33. National Catholic Welfare Conference, "Letter to The Honorable Robert L. Doughton, Chairman of the Committee on Ways and Means," *Hospital Progress* 23 (April 1942): 129; Catholic Hospital Association, "21st and 22nd Resolutions," *Hospital Progress* 23 (October 1942): 307.

34. Shanahan, *The History of the Catholic Hospital Association*, 137.

35. U.S. Bishops, National Catholic War Council, "Program of Social Reconstruction," February 12, 1919, http://www.osjspm.org/majordoc_us_bishops_statements_program_of_social_reconstruction.aspx. Accessed January 27, 2009. The National Catholic War Council was created in 1917 to direct Catholic participation in World War I. See also Jay P. Dolan, *In Search of an American Catholicism: A History of Religion and Culture in Tension* (New York: Oxford University Press, 2002).

36. Alan Derickson, *Health Security for All: Dreams of Universal Health Care in America* (Baltimore: Johns Hopkins University Press, 2005).

37. Donald L. Madison, "From Bismarck to Medicare: A Brief History of Medical Care Payment in America," in *The Social Medicine Reader: Health Policy, Markets, and Medicine*, ed. Jonathan Oberlander, Larry R. Churchill, Sue E. Estroff, Gail E. Henderson, Nancy M. P. King, and Ronald P. Strauss (Durham, N.C.: Duke University Press, 2005), 31–66; Paul Starr, *The Social Transformation of American Medicine* (New York: Basic Books, 1982), 235–310; Joseph S. Ross, "The Committee on the Costs of Medical Care and the History of Health Insurance in the United States," *Einstein Quarterly* 19 (2002): 129–134; Stevens, *In Sickness and in Wealth*, 135; Derickson, *Health Security for All.*

38. Social Security History, http://www.ssa.gov/history/corningchap3.html. Accessed January 23, 2009.

39. "Catholic Viewpoints with Reference to a National Health Program," *Hospital Progress* 24 (November 1943): 329–336.

40. Ibid., 333.

41. Ibid., 331.

42. Shanahan, *The History of the Catholic Hospital Association*, 126–128.

43. Alphonse Schwitalla, "19th Resolution, 1942 CHA Convention," *Hospital Progress* 23 (October 1942): 306–307; and Alphonse Schwitalla, "The Hospital Construction Act," *Hospital Progress* 26 (January 1945): 27–31. This act was an amendment of the Public Health Service Act of 1944 and became Title VI of the act.

44. Alphonse Schwitalla, "Statement by the Rev. Alphonse M. Schwitalla," *Hospital Progress* 26 (March 1945): 77–80.

45. Stevens, *In Sickness and In Wealth*, 217; Kauffman, *A Commitment to Healthcare*, 35.

46. "Catholic Hospitals Plan Wide Expansion," *New York Times*, June 19, 1946; Schwitalla, "The Hospital Construction Act"; Alphonse M. Schwitalla, "The Catholic Hospital Association's Position on the Hospital Construction Act (S.191)," *Hospital Progress* 26 (December 1945): 393; Alphonse M. Schwitalla, "The Hospital Survey and Construction Act (S.191): Introduction," *Hospital Progress* 27 (March 1946): 68. See also Stevens, *In Sickness and in Wealth*, 216–217; Shanahan, *The History of the Catholic Hospital Association*, 129.

47. "The Hill-Burton Act and Civil Rights: Expanding Hospital Care for Black Southerners, 1939–1960," *Journal of Southern History* (November 1, 2006), http://goliath .ecnext.com/coms2/gi_0199–6005519/The-Hill_Burton_Act-and.html. Accessed October 23, 2009.

48. Rheinecker, "Crisis and Reconstruction"; Starr, *The Social Transformation of American Medicine*, 350.

49. *The Official Catholic Directory* (New York: P. J. Kenedy and Sons, 1945); *The Official Catholic Directory* (New York: P. J. Kenedy and Sons, 1950); *The Official Catholic Directory* (New York: P. J. Kenedy and Sons, 1960).

50. Social Security Reform Center—History of Social Security, http://www.social securityreform.org/history/index.cfm. Accessed October 31, 2009.

51. William F. Montavon, "Public Service Rendered by the Voluntary Hospital," *Hospital Progress* 27 (July 1946): 243.

52. Derickson, *Health Security for All*, 96; Daniel Callahan and Angela A. Wasunna, *Medicine and the Market: Equity v. Choice* (Baltimore: Johns Hopkins University Press, 2006); Dolan, *In Search of an American Catholicism*.

53. Report of Management for 1948, UPMC/Mercy Archives.

54. Clayton Knowles, "Catholic Units Hit Federal Care Plan," *New York Times*, April 18, 1949.

55. "American Medical Association Program for the Advancement of Medicine and Public Health," *JAMA* 139, no. 8 (1949): 530.

56. A. M. Mercer, "Inaugural Address," January 1950, n.p., Chancery Correspondence, 1/1/195–12/31/195, Box Mc-M, Archives of the Archdiocese of Chicago, Chicago; "Charities Plan to Fight Federal Welfare Control," *New World*, April 22, 1949. Large hospitals often used black patients for teaching purposes in their clinics.

57. Knowles, "Catholic Units."

58. Callahan and Wasunna, *Medicine and the Market*; Phil Rheinecker, "Catholic Healthcare Enters a New World," in *A Commitment to Healthcare*, ed. Kauffman, 39–44; Stevens, *In Sickness and in Wealth*.

59. *Pacem en Terris*, http://www.vatican.va/holy_father/john_xxiii/encyclicals/ documents/hf_j-xxiii_enc_11041963_pacem_en.html. Accessed January 30, 2009. See also Wills, *Head and Heart*.

60. *Gaudium et Spes*, http://www.vatican.va/archive/hist_councils/ii_vatican_council/ documents/vat-ii_cons_19651207_gaudium-et-spes_en.html. Accessed January 31, 2009; *Populorum Progressio*, http://www.vatican.va/holy_father/paul_vi/encyclicals/ documents/hf_p-vi_enc_26031967_populorum_en.html. Accessed February 19, 2009.

61. *Octogesimus Adveniens,* http://www.osjspm.org/majordoc_octogesima_adveniens _official_text.aspx. Accessed February 19, 2009. For a more thorough discussion of the church's teachings on social justice, see Richard P. McBrien, *Catholicism* (San Francisco: HarperCollins, 1994), 1000–1007; John M. Comey, "The Documents of Vatican II and the Catholic Hospital," *Hospital Progress* 52 (June 1971): 49–56; John T. McGreevy, *Catholicism and American Freedom: A History* (New York: W. W. Norton, 2003); Catholic Health Care in the United States, "Why We Do This: It's Our Mission," http://www.catholichealthcare.us/Our Vision/ActingForReform/WhyWeDoThis.htm. Accessed January 31, 2009.

62. Rosemary Stevens, "Medicare and the Transformation of the Medical Economy," in *Major Problems in the History of American Medicine and Public Health,* ed. John Harley Warner and Janet A. Tighe (Boston: Houghton Mifflin, 2001), 487.

63. Kauffman, *A Commitment to Healthcare,* 50; Thomas F. Casey, "Executive Director's Report," *Hospital Progress* 49 (August 1969): 74. The first woman president of the CHA, a separate office from executive director, was Sister Mary Brigh Cassidy of the Sisters of Saint Francis, in 1967. See also Kauffman, *Ministry and Meaning,* 297–298, 305; Ursula Stepsis and Dolores Liptak, eds., *Pioneer Healers: The History of Women Religious in American Health Care* (New York: Crossroad, 1989), 239–242.

64. Jonathan Engel, *Poor People's Medicine: Medicaid and American Charity Care since 1965* (Durham, N.C.: Duke University Press, 2006), 204–208; Joyce M. Mann, Glenn A. Melnick, Anil Bamezai, and Jack Zwanziger, "A Profile of Uncompensated Hospital Care, 1983–1995," *Health Affairs* 16, no. 4 (July–August 1997): 223–232; Gail R. Wilensky, "Solving Uncompensated Hospital Care: Targeting the Indigent and the Uninsured," *Health Affairs* 3, no. 4 (Winter 1984): 50–62.

65. William E. Kessler, "Healthcare Reform—Entering the Debate," *Health Progress* 73, no. 1 (January–February 1992), http://www.chausa.org/Pub/MainNav/News ?HP/Archive/1992/01JanFeb/Articles/Columns/. Accessed March 4, 2009.

66. Ibid.

67. Stevens, "Medicare and the Transformation of the Medical Economy."

68. Joint Committee on Taxation, "Present Law and Background Relating to the Tax-Exempt Status of Charitable Hospitals, Scheduled for a Hearing before the Senate Committee on Finance, September 13, 2006" (September 12, 2006), http://www.house.gov/jct/x-40-06.pdf. Accessed February 5, 2009. See also James J. McGovern, "Revise or Preserve?" *Health Progress* 73, no. 1 (January–February 1992), http://www.chausa.org/Pub/MainNav/News/HP/Archive/1992/01JanFeb/ Articles/Special. Accessed March 4, 2009.

69. Stevens, *In Sickness and in Wealth,* 345; Phil Rheinecker, "The Threat to Voluntary Hospitals," in Kauffman, *A Commitment to Healthcare,* 53; Emily Friedman, "Taxation as Metaphor," *Health Progress* 73, no. 1 (January–February 1992), http:// www.chausa.org/Pub/MainNav/News/HP/Archive/1992/01JanFeb/Articles/Special. Accessed March 4, 2009.

70. Friedman, "Taxation as Metaphor."

71. This study, by the Prospective Payment Assessment Commission, is reported in J. David Seay, "Community Benefit Prevails," *Health Progress* 73, no. 1 (January–February 1992), http://www.chausa.org/Pub/MainNav/News/HP/Archive/1992/ 01JanFeb/Articles/Special. Accessed March 4, 2009.

72. Arsenio Oloroso Jr., "Hospitals Battle Poverty Care Bill," 1990, copy in ABA.

73. Copy of "Indigent-Care Test Called Counterproductive"; "Bond and Exempt Hospital Lobbies Attack Proposal to Restrict Section 501)(C3) Bonds," *Tax Notes*, October 30, 1989, ADOC; "Tax Changes Could Undermine Indigent Care," *Catholic Health World* 5, no. 22 (November 15, 1989): 1.

74. "Tax Changes Could Undermine Indigent Care."

75. Roger J. Coughlin, Stephen M. Combs, Jean Welter, and Mary E. O'Brien, "Financial Contribution to Community by Catholic Institutions," Catholic Charities brochure, 1988, 76. Rheinecker, "The Threat to the Voluntary Hospital," 54.

77. Angrosino, "The Catholic Church and U.S. Health Care Reform," 7, 12.

78. Joseph Cardinal Bernardin, "Crossroads for Church's Health Care Ministry," *Origins* 22, no. 24 (November 26, 1992): 409–411.

79. Sister Bernice Coreil, "Forging a Future for Catholic Health Care," *Origins* 22, no. 24 (November 26, 1992): 412.

80. Angrosino, "The Catholic Church and U.S. Health Care Reform"; Sister Bernice Coreil, "Values and Vision: CHA's Plan for Healthcare Reform Is Based on Two Unique Perspectives," *Health Progress* 73, no. 2 (March 1992): 34–36; Sister Bernice Coreil, "CHA's Vision of a Redesigned Healthcare System," *Health Progress* 74, no. 4 (May 1993): 12–14.

81. Angrosino, "The Catholic Church and U.S. Health Care Reform"; Coreil, "CHA's Vision."

82. Sister Bernice Coreil, "Healthcare Reform and the Catholic Healthcare Ministry," presented to the Archbishops of the United States 1993 Meeting on Healthcare Reform, May 11, 1993, Chicago, ADOC.

83. U.S. Bishops, "Resolution on Health Care Reform," *Origins* 23, no. 7 (July 1, 1993): 99; Catholic Bishops of the United States, "A Framework for Comprehensive Health Care Reform: Protecting Human Life, Promoting Human Dignity, Pursuing the Common Good," adopted June 18, 1993, ADOC. See also Lartivia A. Hammond and Boxiong Tang, "Indigency, Ethnicity, and Hospital Viability," *Health Progress* 73, no. 10 (December 1992, http://www.chausa.org/Pub/MainNav/News/HP/Archive/1992/12Dec/articles/features/hp9. Accessed January 31, 2009.

84. Derickson, *Health Security for All*.

85. Bishop John Ricard, "Letter to Mrs. Clinton: Reforming Health Care," *Origins* 22 (1993): 782–785.

86. Sister Bernice Coreil, "Statement of The Catholic Health Association of the United States to the President's Health Care Task Force," George Washington University, Washington, D.C., March 29, 1993, ADOC.

87. Gustav Niebuhr, "The Health Care Debate: The Catholic Church; Catholic Leaders' Dilemma: Abortion vs. Universal Care," *New York Times*, August 25, 1994.

88. "Report of Cardinal Hickey on April 29 Meeting with First Lady Hillary Rodham Clinton"; copy of John E. Curley, Jr., to Sister Mary Frances Loftin, September 28, 1993, both in ADOC.

89. "A Proud Moment," *Washington Reform Update*, CHA newsletter, March 31, 1994.

90. "Remarks of Sister Bernice Coreil, the White House," March 23, 1994; CHA News Release, "Catholic Healthcare Providers to Meet with President Clinton," March 18, 1994, both in ADOC.

91. William J. Clinton, "The President's Radio Address," March 26, 1994, http://www.presidency.ucsb.edu/ws/index.php?pid=49880. Accessed February 4, 2009.

92. Transcript, "Organized Religion Raises Moral Issues in Health Care," *Morning Edition*, National Public Radio, March 1994, ADOC.

93. Niebuhr, "The Health Care Debate."

94. "At the Table: CHA, Clintons Meet Privately," *Catholic Health World* 10, no. 17 (September 1, 1994): 1. See also memo, Bill Cox and Jack Bresch to CHA Meeting Participants, re. Private Meeting with the President and First Lady, ADOC.

95. John Michael Cox, "Conscientious Objections to Reform," *Health Progress* 75, no. 2 (March 1994), http://www.chausa.org/Pub/MainNav/News/HP/Archive/1994/ 03Mar. Accessed March 5, 2009.

96. Jonathan Oberlander, "The U.S. Health Care System: On a Road to Nowhere?" in *The Social Medicine Reader: Health Policy, Markets, and Medicine*, ed. Jonathan Oberlander, Larry R. Churchill, Sue E. Estroff, Gail E. Henderson, Nancy M. P. King, and Ronald P. Strauss (Durham, N.C.: Duke University Press, 2005), 5–24.

97. Joseph Cardinal Bernardin, "What Catholics Should Bring to the Health-Care Debate," 1996, http://www.thefreelibrary.com/_/print/PrintArticle.aspx?id=1791 8853. Accessed January 27, 2009.

98. U.S. Conference of Catholic Bishops, "Alert on Medicare" (n.d.), http://www .usccb.org/sdwp/national/medicare.shtml. Accessed December 8, 2009.

99. U.S. Bishops, "Resolution on Health Care Reform."

Chapter 6 — Harassed by Strikes or Threats of Strikes

1. "Union Local 250," *Chronicles*, July 1979, (101) PHO, Box 33, Department of Nursing Service, Strike 1969 folder, SPA.

2. Leon Fink and Brian Greenberg, *Upheaval in the Quiet Zone: A History of Hospital Workers' Union, Local 1199* (Urbana: University of Illinois Press, 1989); Stephen Zuckerman, Gloria Bazzoli, Amy Davidoff, and Anthony LoSasso, "How Did Safety-Net Hospitals Cope in the 1990s?" *Health Affairs* 20, no. 4 (July–August 2001): 159.

3. Colman McCarthy, "Papal Specifics: Commentary," *Washington Post*, September 30, 1979.

4. Fink and Greenberg, *Upheaval*, 106; James A. Gross, ed., *Workers' Rights as Human Rights* (Ithaca, N.Y.: Cornell University Press and ILR Press, 2003); Rosemary Stevens, *In Sickness and in Wealth: American Hospitals in the Twentieth Century* (Baltimore: Johns Hopkins University Press, 1989; repr. 1999), 164.

5. "Significant Dates," 11-TX, Austin Seton, Archives, Daughters of Charity, St. Louis, Mo.

6. Charles R. Morris, *American Catholic: The Saints and Sinners Who Built America's Most Powerful Church* (New York: Vintage Books, 1997); Richard P. McBrien, ed., *The HarperCollins Encyclopedia of Catholicism* (San Francisco: HarperCollins, 1995).

7. Papal Encyclicals Online, http://www.papalencyclicals.net/; and *Laborem Exercens*, http://www.vatican.va/holy_father/john_paul_ii/encyclicals/documents/hf _jp-ii_enc_14091981_laborem-exercens_en.html. Accessed November 29, 2008.

8. *Centesimas Annus*, http://www.vatican.va/holy_father/john_paul_ii/encyclicals/ documents/hf_jp-ii_enc_01051991_centesimus-annus_en.html. Accessed November 29, 2008.

9. Stevens, *In Sickness and in Wealth*, 180.

10. Jean C. Whelan, "Smaller and Cheaper: The Chicago Hourly Nursing Service, 1926– 1957, *Nursing History Review* 10 (2002): 83–108; Philip A. Kalisch and Beatrice J.

Kalisch, *American Nursing: A History*, 4th ed. (Philadelphia: Lippincott Williams and Wilkins, 2004); Barbara Melosh, *"The Physician's Hand": Work Culture and Conflict in American Nursing* (Philadelphia: Temple University Press, 1982); Tom Olson and Eileen Walsh, *Handling the Sick: The Women of St. Luke's and the Nature of Nursing, 1892–1937* (Columbus: Ohio State University Press, 2004).

11. Stevens, *In Sickness and in Wealth*, 164.

12. Susan Reverby, *Ordered to Care: The Dilemma of American Nursing, 1850–1945* (New York: Cambridge University Press, 1987); Melosh, "The Physician's Hand"; Patricia Schechter, "The Labor of Caring: A History of the Oregon Nurses Association," *Oregon Historical Quarterly* 108, no. 1 (Spring 2007), http://www.history cooperative.org/journals/ohq/108.1/schechter.html#FOOT7. Accessed November 24, 2008.

13. Letter from Mary Shea, Seattle, Washington, *RN* 4, no. 7 (1941): 2.

14. B. Jordan, "Labor Gains: Letter to the Editor," *RN* 9, no. 12 (1946): 7; M. E. Wagner, "Labor Opinion: Letter to the Editor," *RN* 10, no. 1 (1946): 14, 16; Beverly Werbes White, "The General Duty Nurse Considers Her Job and Herself," *AJN* [*American Journal of Nursing*] 46, no. 5 (March 1946): 300–301; Reverby, *Ordered to Care*, 197–198.

15. Nurses and Professional Workers Union, Local 126, AFL, Newsletter, 1946.

16. Lyndia Flanagan, *One Strong Voice: The Story of the American Nurses' Association* (Kansas City, Mo.: Lowell Press for the American Nurses' Association, 1976); "The ANA Economic Security Program," *AJN* 47, no. 2 (February 1947): 70–73; Victoria T. Grando, "The ANA's Economic Security Program: The First 20 Years," *Nursing Research* 46, no. 2 (March–April 1997): 111–115.

17. Schechter, "The Labor of Caring"; Flanagan, *One Strong Voice*.

18. Schechter, "The Labor of Caring"; Flanagan, *One Strong Voice*; Reverby, *Ordered to Care*.

19. See "1199: The National Health Care Workers' Union," http://en.wikipedia.org/wiki/Local_1199. Accessed May 16, 2008.

20. The Taft-Hartley Act amended the 1935 National Labor Relations Act. See Anne Zimmerman, "Taft-Hartley Amended: Implications for Nursing," *AJN* 75, no. 2 (February 1975): 284–288; Stevens, *In Sickness and in Wealth*.

21. "Hospitals and Unions—I: General Attitude toward Unions," 4; and "Hospital Labor Unions—II: Meeting the Union Challenge," 1–5, both in (1257) RPP, Box 3, Correspondence, Speeches, Speeches and Writings—Hospitals, SPA.

22. "Hospital Labor Unions—III: If Unions Come," in ibid.

23. See, for example, "34th Resolution, 1942 Convention," *Hospital Progress* 23 (October 1942): 309; "Resolutions, 1948 Convention," *Hospital Progress* 29 (July 1948): 239.

24. John J. Flanagan, "Personnel Problems: A Catholic Approach," *Hospital Progress* 31 (March 1950): 66–68.

25. Monsignor George G. Higgins with William Bole, *Organized Labor and the Church: Reflections of a "Labor Priest"* (New York: Paulist Press, 1993); Christopher J. Kauffman, *Ministry and Meaning: A Religious History of Catholic Health Care in the United States* (New York: Crossroad, 1995).

26. "Celebrating the History of WSNA's First 100 Years," *Washington Nurse*, Spring 2008, n.p. Whereas some nursing organizations organized by alumni associations, those in Washington organized by counties.

27. "Strike," *Chronicles*, August 21, 1958, (101) PHO, SPA. See also "East Bay Hospital Strike Starts Today," *San Francisco Chronicle*, August 21, 1958.

28. "East Bay Hospital Strike Starts Today."

29. Kalisch and Kalisch, *American Nursing*, 432. Founded in 1903 as the California State Nurses Association, the CNA was well known for its long history of advocacy for registered nurses and patients.

30. "Nurses' Crisis," *Chronicles*, July–October 1966, (101) PHO, SPA.

31. "Our Story," from Laurence P. Corbett, Attorney at Law," (101) PHO, SPA.

32. Sister Francis Ignatius, SP, to Mother [Mary Loretta, Provincial Superior], July 2, 1969; "20-Day-Old Bay Nurses' Strike Ends," *Oakland Tribune*, July 2, 1969; "Memorandum to Administrators from Counsel Re. Negotiating Committee Recommended Settlement Associated Hospitals and CAN," June 30, 1969, all in (101) PHO, Box 33, Department of Nursing Service, Strike 1969 folder, SPA.

33. "20-Day-Old Bay Nurses' Strike Ends."

34. "Labor Troubles in Washington"; "Labor Troubles in California"; "Salary Increase," *Chronicles*, July 1, 1966, (56) PSMC Collection, SPA.

35. "Salary Increase."

36. *Chronicles*, 1967, PSMC, SPA.

37. Ibid.

38. U.S. Department of Labor, Bureau of Labor Statistics, *Industry Wage Survey— Hospitals: March 1969* (Washington, D.C.: Government Printing Office, 1971), 1–11. See also Kalisch and Kalisch, *American Nursing*, 432.

39. "Strike Support," *Chronicles*, June 11, 1974, 1974, (101) PHO, Box 33, Department of Nursing Service, Strike 1969 folder, SPA.

40. "Threatened Strike," *Chronicles*, June 5, 1974, in ibid.

41. "The Nurses' Strike—What It's All About," *Oakland Tribune*, June 19, 1974.

42. California Nurses Association, "An Open Letter from the Registered Nurses Represented by CNA," May 30, 1974, (101) PHO, Box 33, Department of Nursing Service, Strike 1974 folder; Peter Stack, "Move Hinted in Nurses' Strike," *San Francisco Chronicle*, June 17, 1974.

43. Editorial, "The Widened Nurses Strike," *San Francisco Daily Review*, June 21, 1974, 20.

44. "Strike Ends," *Chronicles*, June 27, 1974, (101) PHO, Box 33, Department of Nursing Service, Strike 1974 folder, SPA.

45. John G. Kilgour, "Union Organizing Activity in the Hospital Industry," *Hospital and Health Services Administration*, November–December 1984, 81; Zimmerman, "Taft-Hartley Amended"; Taft Hartley Act, http://www.absoluteastronomy.com/topics/Taft-Hartley_Act. Accessed December 15, 2009.

46. Kevin D. O'Rourke, "Christian Responsibility for Labor and Management," *Hospital Progress* 56, no. 7 (July 1975): 63, 64.

47. "Celebrating the History of WSNA's First 100 Years"; Dick Clever, "Hospital Nurses to Strike Today," *Seattle Post-Intelligencer*, July 12, 1976; Lauren Heitmann, "Washington State Nurses Association," June 2002, http://depts.washington.edu/labhist/uwunions/heitmann-wsna.htm. Accessed November 24, 2008.

48. Jerry Bergsman and Al Dieffenbach, "Nurses Post Pickets: Long Strike Feared," *Seattle Times*, July 12, 1976.

49. *Pacer*, July 16 and 30, 1976, (56) PSMC Collection, SPA.

50. Walt Crowley, *To Serve the Greatest Number: A History of Group Health Cooperative of Puget Sound* (Seattle: University of Washington Press, 1996).

51. *Pacer*, July 30, 1976, (56) PSMC Collection, SPA.

52. Ibid., and August 27, 1976.

53. Heitmann, "Washington State Nurses Association."

54. Gregory C. Pope and Terri Menke, "Data Watch," *Health Affairs* 9, no. 4 (Winter 1990): 127–137.

55. "Trends in National and Regional Unionization Rates and in Union versus Nonunion Wages," http://www.piie.com/publications/chapters_preview/352/2iie3411 .pdf. Accessed October 27, 2009. According to the Institute for International Economics, union membership fell by 2.7 million between 1977 and 1987.

56. Ibid.; J. Michael Watt, Robert A. Derzon, Steven C. Renn, Carl J. Schramm, James S. Hahn, and George D. Pillari, "The Comparative Economic Performance of Investor-Owned Chain and Not-for-Profit Hospitals," *New England Journal of Medicine* 314 (1986): 89–96; Raymond J. Baxter and Robert E. Mechanic, "The Status of Local Health Care Safety Nets," *Health Affairs* 16, no. 4 (July–August): 1997): 20; and Zuckerman et al., "How Did Safety-Net Hospitals Cope?" 159.

57. "Nurses' Strike," Letters to the Editor, *Yakima (Wash.) Herald-Republic*, September 21, 1986 (emphasis in original).

58. "Strike Thoughts," Letters to the Editor, *Yakima (Wash.) Herald-Republic*, September 28, 1986; "Nurses' Strike," Letters to the Editor, *Yakima (Wash.) Herald-Republic*, September 23, 1986; "Nurse's Reply," Letters to the Editor, *Yakima (Wash.) Herald-Republic*, September 28, 1986.

59. Sister Dona Taylor to All Employees, July 2 and July 24, 1987; Sister Dona Taylor to Community Advisory Board, Providence Hospital Foundation, Medical Staff, August 4, 1987, all in (101) PHO, SPA.

60. "300 Nurses Go on Strike against Hospital in Oakland," *San Francisco Chronicle*, August 5, 1987.

61. Carolyn Newbergh and Chip Johnson, "Jerry Brown Proclaims Solidarity with Strikers," *Oakland Tribune*, May 28, 1992; National Rainbow Coalition, Inc., Rev. Jesse Jackson, Founder, to the Board of Directors of Summit Medical Center, June 30, 1992, PHO, SPA.

62. "300 Nurses Go on Strike"; Rick Bender, King County Labor Council of Washington, AFL-CIO, to Donald Brennan, Sisters of Providence Corporation, June 29, 1992; CNA to Summit Medical Center Board Members, July 7, 1992, all in (101) Providence Hospital/Summit Medical Center, Strike 1992 folder, PHO, SPA.

63. American Hospital Association, *Hospital Statistics* (Chicago: AHA, 1996–1997).

64. Barbara R. Norrish and Thomas G. Rundall, "Hospital Restructuring and the Work of Registered Nurses," *Milbank Quarterly* 79, no. 1 (2001): 55–79; Linda H. Aiken, Julie Sochalski, and Gerard F. Anderson, "Downsizing the Hospital Nursing Workforce," *Health Affairs* 15, no. 4 (Winter 1996): 88–92.

65. Pope and Menke, "Data Watch"; Watt et al., "The Comparative Economic Performance"; Watt et al., "The Effects of Ownership and Multihospital System Membership"; and B. Langland-Orban, L. Gabenski, and W. B. Bogel, "Differences in Characteristics of Hospitals with Sustained High and Sustained Low Profitability," *Hospital Health Services Administration* 41, no. 3 (1996): 385–399.

66. Lisa Scagliotti, "Nurses Launch Union Drive: Staffers Fear Job Losses as Providence Hospital Reorganizes," *Anchorage Daily News*, May 5, 1994.

67. Mike Hinman, "Nurses Vote on Contract: Providence Plans Striker Substitutes," *Anchorage Daily News*, April 15, 1999; Lisa Demer, "National President Cheers Pickets," *Anchorage Daily News*, April 27, 1999.

68. "PAMC Personnel," *Chronicles*, Providence Medical Center, Anchorage, 1999, (160) Providence Alaska Medical Center, Anchorage, SPA; Eve Rose, "Ready to Walk: Providence Nurses Poised to Strike," *Anchorage Daily News*, April 4, 1999; Eve Rose, "Nurses, Hospital Disagree on What Strike Is About," *Anchorage Daily News*, April 25, 1999.

69. Suzanne Gordon, John Buchanan, and Tanya Bretherton, *Safety in Numbers: Nurse-to-Patient Ratios and the Future of Health Care* (Ithaca, N.Y.: Cornell University Press, 2008).

70. Linda H. Aiken, Herbert L. Smith, and Eileen T. Lake, "Lower Medicare Mortality among a Set of Hospitals Known for Good Nursing Care," *Medical Care* 32, no. 8 (1994): 771–778; Aiken, Sochalski, and Anderson, "Downsizing the Hospital Nursing Workforce"; P. I. Buerhaus and D. O. Staiger, "Managed Care and the Nurse Workforce," *JAMA* 276, no. 18 (1996): 1487–1493; Linda H. Aiken, Sean P. Clarke, Robin B. Cheung, D. M. Sloane, and J. H. Silber, "Education Levels of Hospital Nurses and Patient Mortality," *JAMA* 290 (2003): 1617–1623; Julie A. Sochalski, "Quality of Care, Nurse Staffing, and Patient Outcomes," *Policy, Politics, and Nursing Practice* 2 (2001): 9–18.

71. Mike Hinman, "Nursing Talks to Resume," *Anchorage Daily News*, April 29, 1999; Lisa Demer, "Nurses Approve Contract," *Anchorage Daily News*, May 11, 1999.

72. Kauffman, *Ministry and Meaning*, 121.

73. James C. Robinson and Sandra Dratler, "Corporate Structure and Capital Strategy at Catholic Healthcare West," *Health Affairs* 25, no. 1 (January–February 2006): 134–147.

74. Carl T. Hall, "Catholic Healthcare's Kingdom: CHW Unites 4 Local Affiliate Hospitals for West Bay Region," *San Francisco Chronicle*, July 16, 1996.

75. Hall, "Catholic Healthcare's Kingdom"; Robinson and Dratler, "Corporate Structure."

76. *Examiner* Staff Report, "S.F. Health Care Workers Strike at Two Hospitals," *San Francisco Examiner*, August 13, 1996.

77. Carl T. Hall, "Union Workers Stage Strike at 2 CHW Hospitals," *San Francisco Chronicle*, August 14, 1996; "CHW Hospitals Deliver Union Contract after Short Labor," *San Francisco Business Times*, April 25, 1997; Joanne Spetz, Shannon Mitchell, and Jean Ann Seago, "The Growth of Multihospital Firms in California," *Health Affairs* 19, no. 6 (November–December 2000): 225.

78. Hall, "Catholic Healthcare's Kingdom."

79. William Bole, "Catholic Healthcare West's Organizing Campaign," *Our Sunday Visitor*, November 1998, http://www.catholiclabor.org/gen-art/bole-4.htm. Accessed November 11.

80. Chris Rauber, "Calif. Nurses Strike over Wage Disparity," *Modern Healthcare*, June 29, 1998, http://www.lexisnexis.com/us/lnacademic/frame.do?tokenKey=rsh-20.456250. Accessed December 2, 2008.

81. Spetz, Mitchell, and Seago, "The Growth of Multihospital Firms."

82. James C. Robinson, "Entrepreneurial Challenges to Integrated Health Care," in *Policy Challenges in Modern Health Care*, ed. David Mechanic, Lynn, B. Rogut, David C. Colby, and James R. Knickman (New Brunswick, N.J.: Rutgers University Press, 2005), 53–67.

83. Robinson and Dratler, "Corporate Structure"; Mathew Yi, Michael Dougan, and Pia Sarkar, "Hospital Crisis over Strike," July 6, 2000, *San Francisco Examiner.*

84. George Ramos and Hugo Martin, "Church Role Sought for Southland Labor Disputes," *Los Angeles Times,* September 6, 1999.

85. Linda A. Lotz, "All Religions Believe in Justice," in *Workers' Rights as Human Rights,* ed. Gross, 183–202.

86. Nancy Cleeland, "2 Catholic Hospitals Defeat Union," *Los Angeles Times,* March 25, 2000.

87. Deanna Bellandi and J. Duncan Moore Jr., "SEIU Pressed On," *Modern Healthcare* 30, no. 25 (June 19, 2000): 8.

88. Julie Appleby, "S.F. Hospital Workers to Strike," *USA Today,* July 6, 2000; John M. Glionna and Julie Marquis, "California and the West: 1-Day Strike Hits Hospitals in Bay Area," *Los Angeles Times,* July 7, 2000; J. Duncan Moore, "SEIU Workers Walk Off Job for a Day," *Modern Healthcare* 30, no. 28 (July 10, 2000): 4. See also Alain C. Enthoven and Sara J. Singer, "Managed Competition and California's Healthcare Economy," *Health Affairs* 15, no. 1 (Spring 1996): 40–57.

89. Victoria Colliver, "Hospitals Face 1-Day Strike If No Progress," *San Francisco Examiner,* June 24, 2000.

90. Robinson and Dratler, "Corporate Structure"; Yi, Dougan, and Sarkar, "Hospital Crisis over Strike."

91. Kelly St. John, "9 Hospitals Face Walkout Thursday," *San Francisco Chronicle,* July 3, 2000.

92. Benjamin Pimentel, Kelly St. John, and Chuck Squatriglia, "Both Sides Claim Victory in 1-Day Hospital Walkout," *San Francisco Chronicle,* July 7, 2000; Carol Ness and Pia Sarkar, "Hospital Workers Returning to Jobs after 1-Day Strike," *San Francisco Examiner,* July 7, 2000.

93. Benjamin Pimentel and Kelly St. John, "Future Hospital Strikes Worry Health Official," *San Francisco Chronicle,* August 3, 2000.

94. "Hospital Workers Strike," *Silicon Valley/San Jose Business Journal,* October 25, 2000.

95. Arthur Jones, "Catholic Hospital Organization Signs Accord with Union," *National Catholic Reporter,* 2002, http://natcath.org/NCR_Online/archives2/2001b/042001/042001h.htm. Accessed October 21, 2008; George G. Higgins, "The Catholic Hospital Leadership of Women," *Catholic-Labor Network,* May 8, 2000, http://www.catholiclabor.org/higgins/higgins-67.htm. Accessed November 19, 2008.

96. George G. Higgins, "The Challenge for Some Catholic Hospitals," *Catholic-Labor Network,* March 29, 1999, http://www.catholiclabor.org/higgins/higgins-38.htm. Accessed November 19, 2008; Economic Justice for All: Pastoral Letter on Catholic Social Teaching and the U.S. Economy, http://www.osjspm.org/economic_justice_for_all.aspx. Accessed December 2, 2008.

97. Jones, "Catholic Hospital Organization."

98. United Conference of Catholic Bishops, "A Fair and Just Workplace: Principles and Practices for Catholic Health Care," http://www.usccb.org/sdwp/national/place.shtml. Accessed October 21, 2008.

99. Ibid.

100. Fact Sheet: "A Fair and Just Workplace: Principles and Practices for Catholic Health Care," August 26, 1999, http://www.usccb.org/sdwp/national/factsheet.shtml. Accessed October 21, 2008. See also George G. Higgins, "Justice in Catholic Hospitals, Yes, and All Catholic Institutions," January 31, 2000,

Catholic-Labor Network, http://www.catholiclabor.org/higgins/higgins-61.htm. Accessed November 19, 2008.

101. Sister Mary Roch Rocklage, "A Just and Fair Workplace: Principles and Practices for Catholic Health Care," August 26, 1999, http://www.catholiclabor.org/hospital/rocklage.htm. Accessed November 19, 2008.

102. National Interfaith Committee for Worker Justice, "Guidelines for Unions and Management of Religiously Sponsored Healthcare Institutions," Chicago, Illinois, March 1999, http://www.workplacefairness.org/groups-nicwj_home. Accessed November 19, 2008.

103. Jerry Filteau, "Catholic Health System, Union Set Expedited Election Rules," *Catholic-Labor Network*, April 10, 2001, http://www.catholiclabor.org/hospital/chw-seiu.htm. Accessed November 19, 2008.

104. Noted in Jones, "Catholic Hospital Organization."

105. Don Lee, "Catholic Healthcare West, Union Reach Accords," *Los Angeles Times*, April 26, 2002; Simon J. Craddock Lee, "Charism and Community: Catholic Women Religious and the Corporate Commitment to Healthcare," http://www.religionandsocialpolicy.org/docs/events2003_spring_research_conference/lee.pdf. Accessed November 19, 2008. See also Bernita McTernan, taped telephone interview by author, March 9, 2009.

106. Jones, "Catholic Hospital Organization."

107. Sister Patricia A. Talone, RN, PhD, http://www.chausa.org/Talone_Sr_Patricia. Accessed October 31, 2009.

108. Sister Patricia Talone, "Labor and Catholic Health Care," *Health Progress* 83, no. 2 (March–April 2002): 36–38, 60.

109. Ibid. See also Thomas Bokenkotter, *A Concise History of the Catholic Church* (New York: Image Books, Doubleday, 1990); Dolan, *In Search of an American Catholicism*.

110. Talone, "Labor and Catholic Health Care."

111. Ibid.

112. Noted in Arthur Jones, "Catholic Aim: Aid Poor, Survive," *National Catholic Reporter*, June 6, 2003, 3–4. See also Rocklage, "A Just and Fair Workplace."

113. "U.S. Bishops Issue Guidelines for Catholic Health Care-Labor Disputes," Catholic News Agency, http://www.catholicnewsagency.com/new.php?n=16362. Accessed December 14, 2009.

114. McTernan interview; see also Jones, "Catholic Hospital Organization"; Higgins, "The Catholic Hospital Leadership of Women;" Sister Helene Lentz, CSJ, e-mail correspondence with author, November 3, 2009.

115. Brendan Doherty and Kathy Robertson, "Sisters Call Back Seven CHW Hospitals," *Sacramento Business Journal*, May 25, 2001.

116. Joe Marti, "Hospital Break-Up: Daughters of Charity Go It Alone," *San Francisco Faith* (March 2002), http://www.sffaith.com/ed/articles/2002/0302jm.htm. Accessed October 27, 2009.

117. McTernan interview; Robinson and Dratler, "Corporate Structure," 146.

Chapter 7 — Practical Solutions to Complicated Problems

1. Lucette Lagnado, "Religious Practice: Their Role Growing, Catholic Hospitals Juggle Doctrine and Medicine," *Wall Street Journal*, February 4, 1999.

2. Ibid.

3. Letters to the Editor, *Wall Street Journal*, February 23, 1999.

4. Joyce Gelb and Colleen J. Shogan, "Community Activism in the USA: Catholic Hospital Mergers and Reproductive Access," *Social Movement Studies* 4, no. 3 (December 2005): 209–229; Matt McDonald, "The Limits of Cooperation," *Catholic World News*, October 1, 2001, http://www.catholicculture.org/news/features/index.dfm?recnum=20540. Accessed March 28, 2009.

5. "Is There a Common Ground: Affiliations between Catholic and Non-Catholic Health Care Providers and the Availability of Reproductive Health Services?" #1322, Henry J. Kaiser Family Foundation, November 1997. The table is based on data from the American Hospital Association, *Modern Healthcare*, and the Catholic Health Association, http://search.kff.org/gsaresults/search?site=KFForgno pdfs&filter=0&output=xml_no_dtd&client=kff&sp=kff&getfields=*&q=Is%20 There%20a%20Common%20Ground:%20Affiliations%20between%20Catholic %20and%20Non-Catholic%20Health%20Care%20Providers%20and%20the%20 Availability%20of%20Reproductive%20Health%20Services?"%20&no_pdf=1. Accessed April 13, 2009.

6. John M. Haas, "Reproductive Technologies," in *Urged On by Christ: Catholic Health Care in Tension with Contemporary Culture, Proceedings of the Twenty-First Workshop for Bishops*, ed. Edward J. Furton (Philadelphia: National Catholic Bioethics Center, 2007), 35.

7. David F. Kelly, *Contemporary Catholic Health Care Ethics* (Washington, D.C.: Georgetown University Press, 2004), 9n1.

8. John T. McGreevy, "Catholics in America: Antipathy and Assimilation," in *American Catholics, American Culture: Tradition and Resistance*, vol. 2, *American Catholics in the Public Square*, ed. Margaret O'Brien Steinfels (Lanham, Md.: Rowman and Littlefield, 2004), 3–26; Kathleen M. Joyce, "Medicine, Markets, and Morals: Catholic Hospitals and the Ethics of Abortion in Early 20th-Century America," Cushwa Center for the Study of American Catholicism, University of Notre Dame, Working Paper Series 29, no. 2 (South Bend, Ind.: Cushwa Center, Fall 1997).

9. McGreevy, "Catholics in America"; Kristin Luker, *Abortion and the Politics of Motherhood* (Berkeley: University of California Press, 1984), 59–61; Casti Connubi, http://www.vatican.va/holy_father/pius_xi/encyclicals/documents/hf_p-xi_enc _31121930_casti-connubii_en.html. Accessed April 13, 2009.

10. Michael P. Bourke, "A Surgical Code," *Hospital Progress* 1 (May 1920): 36; Richard P. McBrien, ed., *Encyclopedia of Catholicism* (San Francisco: HarperCollins, 1995), 6.

11. McGreevy, "Catholics in America"; Luker, *Abortion and the Politics of Motherhood*.

12. McGreevy, "Catholics in America"; Luker, *Abortion and the Politics of Motherhood*; Leslie Woodcock Tentler, ed., *The Church Confronts Modernity: Catholicism since 1950 in the U.S., Ireland, and Quebec* (Washington, D.C.: Catholic University of America Press, 2007); Ellen Carol Dubois and Lynn Dumenil, *Through Women's Eyes: An American History with Documents* (Boston: Bedford/St. Martin's, 2005).

13. Pellegrino, "Catholic Health Care Ministry and Contemporary Culture: The Growing Divide," 13–30.

14. McGreevy, "Catholics in America," 16; Leslie Woodcock Tentler, *Catholics and Contraception: An American History* (Ithaca, N.Y.: Cornell University Press, 2004). See also "The Sanctity of Human Life," http://www.secondexodus.com/

html/vaticandocs/volumedirectories/sanctityofhumanlife.htm. Accessed December 16, 2009.

15. Tentler, *Catholics and Contraception*. See also *Humanae Vitae*, Encyclical of Pope Paul VI on the Regulation of Birth (1968), http://www.vatican.va/holy_father/ paul_vi/encyclicals/documents/hf_p-vi_enc_25071968_humanae-vitae_en.html. Accessed January 15, 2008.

16. William V. D'Antonio, James D. Davidson, and Dean R. Hoge, *American Catholics: Gender, Generation, and Commitment* (Walnut Creek, Calif.: Alta Mira Books, 2004); James D. Davidson, *The Search for Common Ground* (Huntington, Ind.: Our Sunday Visitor Books, 1997).

17. Pellegrino, "Catholic Health Care Ministry," 19, 21.

18. Joseph Cardinal Bernardin, *Consistent Ethic of Life* (Kansas City, Mo.: Sheed and Ward, 1988), http://archives.archchicago.org/JCBpdfs/JCBathealthcarereform.pdf.

19. "Coalition of Nuns Criticizes Bishops' Stand on Abortion," *New York Times*, October 11, 1984; Kenneth Briggs, "Nuns, Expressing Dismay, Ponder Vatican Threat," *New York Times*, December 20, 1984; UPI, "Around the Nation: 11 Nuns Deny Statement by Vatican on Abortion," *New York Times*, July 25, 1986; Roberto Suro, "Superiors Refuse to Dismiss Nuns in Abortion Case," *New York Times*, June 6, 1988; Francis Kissling, "The Best and the Brightest of the Catholic Bad Girls," http://www.awid.org/Issues-and-Analysis/Library/The-Best-and-the-Brightest-of-the-Catholic-Bad-Girls. Accessed May 19, 2010.

20. Haas, "Reproductive Technologies," 37.

21. McBrien, *Encyclopedia*, 1, 105; Kevin D. O'Rourke, Thomas Kopfensteiner, and Ron Hamel, "A Brief History: A Summary of the Development of the *Ethical and Religious Directives for Catholic Health Care Services*," *Health Progress* 82, no. 6 (November–December 2001), http://www.chausa.org/Pub/MainNav/News/HP/ Archive/2001/11NovDec/Articles/Feature. Accessed December 30, 2007. See also Marin L. Cook, "Guest Editorial: Reproductive Technologies and the Vatican," Markkula Center for Applied Ethics, http://www.scu.edu/ethics/publications/ iie/v1n3/homepage.html. Accessed February 7, 2009.

22. Sister Jean deBlois and Reverend Kevin D. O'Rourke, "Care for the Beginning of Human Life," *Health Progress* 76, no. 7 (September–October 1995). http://www .chausa.org/Pub/MainNav/News/HP/Archive/1995/09SeptOct/Articles/Features. Accessed August 24, 2007.

23. Charles J. Barnett, Memo, May 4, 1995; *Seton Leader Letter*, A Seton Network Special Issue, May 4, 1995, both in AHC.

24. Charles J. Barnett to David B. Coats, January 13, 1995; Memo, January 19, 1995; Charles J. Barnett to David B. Coats and Jesus Garza, January 31, 1995; Memorandum to Mayor and Council Members from Jesus Garza, City Manager, May 3, 1995, all in AHC.

25. U.S. Conference of Catholic Bishops, *Ethical and Religious Directives for Catholic Health Care Services* (Washington, D.C.: USCCB, 1994). See also O'Rourke, Kopfensteiner, and Hamel, "A Brief History"; Rachel Benson Gold, "Hierarchy Crackdown Clouds Future of Sterilization, EC Provision at Catholic Hospitals," *Guttmacher Report on Public Policy* 5, no. 2 (May 2002), http://www.guttmacher .org/pubs/tgr/05/2/gr050211.html. Accessed December 30, 2007. The Alan Guttmacher Institute is a New York–based think tank on reproductive issues.

26. *Seton Leader Letter*.

27. Liz Bucar, "Caution: Catholic Health Restrictions May Be Hazardous to Your Health," http://www.catholicsforchoice.org/topics/healthcare/documents/1998 cautioncatholichealthrestrictions.pdf. Accessed January 15, 2008; Deanna Bellandi, "CHA Counterattacks Study on Mergers," *Modern Healthcare* 29, no. 19 (May 10, 1999): 14; "Report of the Task Force on Ethical and Religious Directives," *Linacre Quarterly* (May 2005): 174.

28. Bucar, "Caution;" Bellandi, "CHA Counterattacks;" "Report of the Task Force."

29. Daniel Callahan and Angela A. Wasunna, *Medicine and the Market: Equity v. Choice* (Baltimore: Johns Hopkins University Press, 2006).

30. Rachel Benson Gold, "Contraceptive Coverage: Toward Ensuring Access While Respecting Conscience," *Guttmacher Report on Public Policy* 1, no. 6 (December 1998). http://www.guttmacher.org/pubs/tgr/01/6/gr010601.html. Accessed August 23, 2007. Gloria Feldt, "Congress Is Foiling Americans' Desire for Reproductive Choice," *USA Today*, May 1, 1999; "Baby Boom: American Anti-Abortion Politics Blocks Family Planning Funding around the World," *emagazine.com* 9, no. 6 (November–December 1998), http://www.emagazine.com/view/?822andsrc=. Accessed August 23, 2007. Rosemary Radford Ruether, "Women, Reproductive Rights and the Catholic Church," Catholics for a Free Choice, May 2006, http://www.catholicsforchoice.org/print.asp. Accessed August 24, 2007.

31. Essay noted in Patricia Byrne, "Diminishment, Delusion, Discovery, 1970–," in *Transforming Parish Ministry: The Changing Roles of Catholic Clergy, Laity, and Women Religious*, ed. Jay P. Dolan, R. Scott Appleby, Patricia Byrne, and Debra Campbell (New York: Crossroad, 1990), 182 (emphasis in original).

32. Memo re. Brackenridge Hospital Governance/Austin Hospital Authority; John Nuveen and Co., Inc., "Nuveen Mergers and Acquisitions, Introduction to Services for Seton Medical Center," both in AHC.

33. *Seton Leader Letter.*

34. "Hospitals Are Still Deflecting Emergency Patients, Group Says," *New York Times*, October 30, 1994. The study was done by the Public Citizen Health Research Group.

35. A. B. Bindman, D. Keane, and N. Lurie, "A Public Hospital Closes: Impact on Patients' Access to Care and Health Status," *JAMA* 264, no. 22 (1990), http://jama.ama-assn.org/cgi/content/abstract/264/22/2899. Accessed January 1, 2008.

36. Louisa C. Brinsmade, "Brack Gets Religion," n.d., AHC; Mike Todd, "City Council Approves Brackenridge Lease," *Austin American-Statesman*, May 26, 1995.

37. In addition to Monsignor Broussard, the ethicists included Reverend Gerard Magill, PhD, associate professor of theology at St. Louis University; Reverend Dennis Brodeur, senior vice president for stewardship for the Franciscan Sisters of Mary Health Systems in St. Louis; and Dominican Fathers Kevin O'Rourke and Benedict Ashley, who had coauthored a two-volume theological analysis of health care ethics.

38. Monsignor William L. Broussard to Mr. James Kramer, April 24, 1995, AHC.

39. The principle of cooperation in the 1994 *Ethical and Religious Directives* was in line with the Congregation for the Defense of the Faith's statement on sterilization, *Quaecumque Sterilizatio.*

40. Kelly, *Contemporary Catholic Health Care Ethics*, 256.

41. Gerard Magill, "Seton/Brackenridge Lease Agreement and the Principle of Material Cooperation," June 28, 1995, 13–14 (emphasis in original), AHC.

42. Ibid., 19–20. Physicians were independent practitioners, not city or Seton employees.

43. Richard Daly, "John McCarthy," *Brief Biographies of the First Two Directors: The Texas Catholic Conference, 1963–1979* (Austin: Texas Catholic Conference, 1979), AHC; Bishop John McCarthy, taped interview by author, December 5, 2007, Austin, Texas.

44. McCarthy interview.

45. Kathryn Saenz Duke, "Hospitals in a Changing Health Care System," *Health Affairs* 15, no. 2 (Summer 1996): 53.

46. A 1999 study verified this concern and showed that after conversions of hospitals to for-profit status, communities lose significant services and resources, which can lead to decreased access to care. See S.Y.D. Lee and J. A. Alexander, "Managing Hospitals in Turbulent Times: Do Organizational Changes Improve Hospital Survival?" *Health Services Research* 34, no. 4 (1999): 923–944.

47. Ibid.; John McCarthy, Bishop of Austin, to Sister Patricia Elder, D.C., Chair Seton Medical Center Board of Trustees, May 18, 1995, AHC.

48. Charles M. Wilson to His Eminence Joseph Cardinal Ratzinger, May 17, 1995, AHC; McCarthy interview. A later letter from Concerned Catholics of Austin to Charles J. Barnett, May 27, 2997, AHC, also made these charges.

49. McBrien, *Encyclopedia.*

50. McCarthy interview; Memo to Seton Board of Trustees, July 30, 1998; Kim Sue Lia Perkes, "Vatican Questions Austin Bishop over Brackenridge," and "Chronology of a Controversy," *Austin American-Statesman*, July 30, 1998.

51. McCarthy interview.

52. Perkes, "Vatican Questions Austin Bishop."

53. Memo, Pat Hayes to Seton Board of Trustees, July 30, 1998, AHC.

54. Dennis J. Eike to Sister Marie Therese Sedgwick, July 7, 1997, AHC.

55. Paul Likoudis, "Chancery Documents Indicate Bishop Deceived Vatican," *The Wanderer*, n.d., AHC.

56. Editorial, "Bishop Needs Support," *Austin American-Statesman*, July 31, 1998. According to Jay P. Dolan, the hierarchical nature of the church versus its communal character has been a contentious issue for American Catholics since the early 1800s. See Jay P. Dolan, *The American Catholic Experience: A History from Colonial Times to the Present* (Notre Dame, Ind.: University of Notre Dame Press, 1992).

57. Kim Sue Lia Perkes, "Seton, Austin, Working on Brackenridge Lease," *Austin American-Statesman*, August 20, 1998.

58. Ibid.; Kim Sue Lia Perkes and Mary Ann Roser, "For Seton, a Debate of Church vs. Choice," *Austin American-Statesman*, December 31, 2000.

59. Kim Sue Lia Perkes, "Bishops to Weigh Hospital Services," *Austin American-Statesman*, October 26, 2000. See also Frances Kissling, "Is There Life after *Roe*? How to Think about the Fetus," *Conscience: The News Journal of Catholic Opinion*, Winter 2004–2005, http://www.catholicsforchoice.org/print/asp. Accessed January 2, 2008.

60. Kelly, *Contemporary Catholic Health Care Ethics*, 121. U.S. Conference of Catholic Bishops, *Ethical and Religious Directives for Catholic Health Care Services*, 4th ed., June 15, 2001; see also O'Rourke, Kopfensteiner, and Hamel, "A Brief History."

61. Noted in Gayle White and Mary Ann Roser, "Catholic Bishops Adopt Policies That Reinforce Beliefs," *Austin American-Statesman*, June 16, 2001.

62. "Naked City," *Austin Chronicle*, June 8, 2001.

63. Mary Ann Roser and Kim Sue Lia Perkes, "Seton to Limit Some Services at Brack," *Austin American-Statesman*, June 8, 2001.

64. Quoted in Mary Ann Roser and Kim Sue Lia Perkes, "City May Run Birth Control at Brack," *Austin American-Statesman*, August 22, 2001.

65. Gold, "Hierarchy Crackdown." Before September 1998, no EC product had been approved, labeled, and marketed in the United States, and emergency hormonal contraception was available only through off-label use of oral contraceptive pills. Off-label use of approved medications was legal, and some hospital emergency rooms and family-planning clinics provided women with EC in this way. See also "Emergency Contraception Use Up—New ECP Arrives," *Contraceptive Technology Update 20*, no. 9 (1999): 108–109.

66. U.S. Conference of Catholic Bishops, *Ethical and Religious Directives*, 2001; Catholics for a Free Choice, "The Facts about Catholic Health Care in the United States," *Catholic Health Care Update* (Washington, D.C.: Catholics for a Free Choice, September 2005), 4; Catholics for a Free Choice, "Second Chance Denied: Emergency Contraception in Catholic Hospital Emergency Rooms," 2002, http://www.catholics forchoice.org/topics/healthcare/documents/2002secondchancedenied_001.pdf. Accessed May 13, 2009.

67. Gold, "Hierarchy Crackdown"; Suzanne Batchelor, "Clash and Compromise: Ethics at Issue When Public Hospital Is Put into Catholic Hands," *National Catholic Reporter*, July 4, 2003, www.findarticles.com/p/articles/mi_m1141/is_33_39/ai_105480211/print. Accessed August 23, 2007.

68. "Letters," *Austin American-Statesman*, December 21, 2001, n.p.

69. Andrew Park, "Seton Extending Health-Care Reach," *Austin American-Statesman*, October 6, 1998.

70. Quoted in "Naked City," n.p.

71. McCarthy interview.

72. Alan M. Zukerman, "A Promising Form of Consolidation: Joint Operating Agreements Are Gaining Popularity," *Health Progress* 81, no. 4 (July–August, 2000): 14–16.

73. Moral Sterility, http://www.osv.com/tabid/7621/itemid/3842/In-Focus-Moral-steriltiy.aspx. Accessed December 15, 2009.

74. Peter J. Cataldo and John M. Haas, "Institutional Cooperation: The ERDs," *Health Progress* 83, no. 6 (November–December 2002). https://mail.nursing.upenn.owa/?ae=Itemanda=Openandt=IPM.Noteandid=RgAAAAC%2b. Accessed March 31, 2009.

75. Catholics for a Free Choice, "The Facts about Catholic Health Care in the United States"; Rachel Benson Gold, "Advocates Work to Preserve Reproductive Health Care Access When Hospitals Merge," *Guttmacher Report on Public Policy* 3, no. 2 (April 2000), http://www.guttmacher.org/pubs/tgr/03/2/gr030203.html. Accessed September 23, 2008. Catholics for a Free Choice, "Second Chance Denied."

76. Gelb and Shogan, "Community Activism."

77. Ibid.

78. Patricia Donovan, "Hospital Mergers and Reproductive Health Care," *Family Planning Perspectives* 28, no. 6 (November–December 1996): 281–284.

79. James C. Capretta, "Health Care with a Conscience," *New Atlantis*, Fall 2008, 76. Capretta is a fellow at the Ethics and Public Policy Center. In the mid-1990s, he worked for the Catholic Health Association as a government relations officer.

80. Chuck Moody, "'60 Minutes' Disappoints Mercy Health CEO," *Pittsburgh Catholic*, December 15, 2000, 3; and "Letters: '60 Minutes' Segment One-Sided," *Pittsburgh Catholic*, December 29, 2000, n.p.

81. "Naked City."

82. Lagnado, "Religious Practice."

Chapter 8 — *S* Stands for "Sister," Not "Stupid"

1. Sister Felice Sauers, taped telephone interview with author, August 17, 2009. Sister Felice has been codirector of Mercy Association in Burlingame, California, and has served on several Catholic hospital boards.

2. Clarke E. Cochran, "Pope Benedict XVI's New Encyclical: Implications for Catholic Health Care," *Health Progress* 90, no. 5 (September–October 2009), http://www.chausa.org/Pub/MainNav/News/HP/Archive/2009Sept. Accessed October 29, 2009.

3. Kevin O'Rourke, "Are Catholic Acute Care Hospitals Worth the Effort?" http://www.salus-sofia.net/contributions/orourke/catholic-acute-care-hospitals-worth-the-effort. Accessed February 14, 2009.

4. Mary Maurita Sengelaub, "Catholic Health Care Systems: A Sign of the Times," *Hospital Progress* 59, no. 11 (November 1978): 56.

5. Patricia Wittberg, *From Piety to Professionalism—and Back? Transformations of Organized Religious Virtuosity* (New York: Lexington Books, 2006); Doris Gottemoeller, "Institutions without Sisters," *Review for Religious* 50 (1991): 564–571. Sister Doris served as chair of the CHA Board of Trustees from 1998 to 1999.

6. Richard A. McCormick, "The End of Catholic Hospitals?" *America* 179, no. 1 (July 4, 1998): 5–6; Joseph Cardinal Bernardin, "A Sign of Hope: A Pastoral Letter on Healthcare" (Chicago: Archdiocese of Chicago, October 18, 1995); Sister Karin Dufault, "Offering a Flickering Light: How Caregivers Contribute to Atmospheres of Hope," *Health Progress* 89, no. 3 (May–June 2008): 57–61.

7. Bernita McTernan, taped telephone interview with author, March 9, 2009; Gottemoeller, "Institutions without Sisters."

8. McTernan interview.

9. Sister Doris Gottemoeller, "Preserving Our Catholic Identity," *Health Progress* 80, no. 3 (May–June 1999), http://www.chausa.org/Pub/MainNav/News/HP/Archive/1999/05MayJune/Articles/Feature. Accessed May 15, 2009. See also Bruce Japsen, "Columbia's Big Catholic Deal Faces Scrutiny," *Modern Healthcare* 25, no. 21 (1995): 2–4, 10.

10. Sengelaub, "Catholic Health Care Systems"; Sister Marie Damian Glatt and Gerard Magill, "Organizational Decision Making for Catholic Health Care Partnerships," *Health Care Ethics* 8, no. 4 (Fall 2000) (emphasis in original), http://hce.slu.edu/hceusa/fall_2000_1.html. Accessed June 9, 2009.

11. Gottemoeller, "Institutions without Sisters," 566.

12. McTernan interview.

13. Sister Helene Lentz, e-mail communication with author, November 3, 2009.

14. The Ministries of Pittsburgh Mercy, http://www.pmhs.org/. Accessed July 8, 2009.

15. McTernan interview.

16. Alexian Brothers Medical Center, http://www.alexianbrothershealth.org/index
    .aspx. Accessed July 8, 2009.
17. AHA News, http://www.ahanews.com/ahanews_app/jsp/display.jsp?dcrpath=AHA
    NEWS/AHANewsArticle/data/AHA_News_050919_Sister_Carolanddomain=AHA
    NEWS. Accessed June 24, 2009.
18. Ibid.; McTernan interview.
19. Barbra Mann Wall, *Unlikely Entrepreneurs: Catholic Sisters and the Hospital Mar-
    ketplace, 1865–1925* (Columbus: Ohio State University Press, 2005).
20. Stacey Burling, "Catholic Health East Names a New Leader," http://www.philly
    .com/philly/business/20091216_Catholic_Health_East_names_a_new_leader
    .html. Accessed December 17, 2009.
21. AHA News, http://www.ahanews.com/ahanews_app/jsp/display.jsp?dcrpath=AHA
    NEWS/AHANewsArticle/data/AHA_News_050919_Sister_Carolanddomain=AHA
    NEWS. Accessed December 17, 2009.
22. Sister Sheila Lyne, taped telephone interview with author, May 29, 2009.
23. See, for example: Pittsburgh Mercy—History, http://www.pmhs.org/mccauley-
    ministries/mission-values-and-vision.aspx. Accessed December 12, 2009.
24. Charles L. Harper and Bryan F. LeBeau, "Social Change and Religion in America:
    Thinking beyond Secularization," http://are.as.wvu.edu/sochange.htm. Accessed
    April 2, 2007.
25. Kevin O'Rourke, "Are Catholic Acute Care Hospitals Worth the Effort?" http://
    www.salus-sofia.net/contributions/orourke/catholic-acute-care-hospitals-worth
    -the-effort. Accessed February 14, 2009; Clarke E. Cochran and Kenneth R. White,
    "Does Catholic Sponsorship Matter? *Health Progress* 83, no. 1 (January–February
    2002), http://www.chausa.org/cgi-bin.MsmGo.exe?grab_id=0andpage-id=7554and
    query=study%2002. Accessed March 31, 2009. See also Advocacy/Policy Briefs,
    http://www.chausa.org/Pub/MainNav/Advocacy/policybriefs/. Accessed July 17,
    2008.
26. Catholic Health Association of the United States, American Hospital Association,
    and Federation of American Hospitals, "Statement about Agreement with White
    House and Senate Finance Committee on Health Reform," July 8, 2009, http://www
    .aha.org/aha/press-release/2009/090708-jointst-covreform.pdf. Accessed July 8,
    2009.
27. Health Care Letter by U.S. Conference of Catholic Bishops to the Senate, Novem-
    ber 20, 2009, http://www.usccb.org/sdwp/national/2009–11–20-ltr-usccb-health-
    care-to-senate.pdf. Accessed July 8, 2009; David D. Kirkpatrick and Robert Pear,
    "A Victory in Health Care Vote for Opponents of Abortion," *New York Times*,
    November 9, 2009; "Catholic Health Association Reaffirms Long-Standing Com-
    mitment to Reform Health Care but Waits to Endorse Any Specific Bill," http://
    www.prnewswire.com/news-releases/catholic-health-association-reaffirms
    -long-standing-commitment.html; Kathleen Gilbert, "Catholic Organizations'
    Support for Health Care Reform Follows the Money Trail," http://www.lifesite-
    news.com/ldn/2009/aug/09080705.html. Accessed December 20, 2009.
28. Opinion, http://www.missoulian.com/news/opinion/mailbag/article_7cd4873e-
    eb1d-11de-8835–001cc4c03286.html; Sister Carol Keehan, http://odeo.com/
    episodes/25004551-Health-Care-Reform-Debate-Raymond-Arroyo-with-Sr-Carol-
    Keehan-of-CHA-and-Judie-Brown-of-ALL; and Bishop Nickless: No Health Care

Reform Better than Wrong Health Care Reform, http://www.catholic.org/politics/story.php?id=34271. Accessed December 17, 2009.

29. Sister Carol Keehan, http://odeo.com/episodes/25004551-Health-Care-Reform-Debate-Raymond-Arroyo-with-Sr-Carol-Keehan-of-CHA-and-Judie-Brown-of-ALL (emphasis in original). Accessed December 17, 2009. Catholic Health Association of the United States, "Reasons Health Reform Would Be Beneficial," http://www.chausa.org/Pub/MainNav/ourcommitments/Health+Reform/Reasons.htm. Accessed January 1, 2010.

30. Background: Hyde/Weldon Conscience Protection Amendment in the Labor/HHS Appropriations Bill, http://www.usccb.org/prolife/issues/abortion/h-backgrounder.pdf. Accessed January 1, 2010. John Patton Fortuno, "The Weldon Amendment: The Ongoing Restrictions on a Woman's Right to Choose," April 4, 2006, http://law.bepress.com/expresso/eps/1243/. Accessed December 17, 2009. See also Heather D. Boonstra, "The Heart of the Matter: Public Funding of Abortion for Poor Women in the United States," *Guttmacher Policy Review* 10, no 1 (Winter 2007), http://www.guttmacher.org/pubs/gpr/10/1/gpr100112.html. Accessed January 1, 2010.

31. Marie T. Hilliard, "Contraceptive Mandates and the Avoidance of Culpable Negligence," in *Urged On by Christ*, ed. Furton, 127–141. See also Fortuno, "The Weldon Amendment"; and Boonstra, "The Heart of the Matter." Women's rights activists challenged the Hyde and Weldon Amendments as discriminatory, particularly against low-income women, since the amendments primarily affected Medicaid services to the poor.

32. "Catholic Bishops Shape Health Care Bill," http://www.msnbc.msn.com/id/33852621/ns/politics-health_care_reform/. Accessed December 20, 2009.

33. Ibid.

34. Kirkpatrick and Pear, "A Victory in Health Care Vote."

35. David D. Kirkpatrick, "Catholic Group Supports Senate on Abortion Aid," *New York Times*, December 25, 2009.

36. Nancy Frazier O'Brien, "'Not a Shred of Disagreement' between CHA, Bishops on Health Reform," *Catholic News Service*, December 28, 2009. http://www.catholic-news.com/data/stories/cns/0905688.htm. Accessed January 1, 2010.

37. Mitchell Landsberg, "Nuns in U.S. Back Healthcare Bill Despite Catholic Bishops' Opposition," www.latimes.com/om/features/health/la-na-healthcare-nuns18-2010 mar18,0,7687394.story. Accessed March 18, 2010.

38. Sister Carol Keehan to Representative, March 11, 2010, www.chausa.org. Accessed March 18, 2010. See also Sister Carol Keehan, "The Time Is Now for Health Reform." http://www.chausa.org/Sr._Carol_Column/. Accessed March 22, 2010.

39. Network: A National Catholic Social Justice Lobby, "Catholic Sisters Support Passage of Healthcare Bill," http://www.networklobby.org/press/3–17–10Healthcare SistersLetter.htm. Accessed March 18, 2010.

40. USCCB, "President of U.S. Bishops Says Cost Is Too High, Loss Is Too Great for Health Care Bill Not to Be Revised," news release, http://www.usccb.org/comm/archives/2010/10–043.shtml. Accessed March 18, 2010.

41. Landsberg, "Nuns in U.S."; and Karoli, "Catholic Nuns Endorse HCR in Defiance of Bishops' Mandate," http://crooksandliars.com/node/35689/print. Accessed March 18, 2010.

42. I Can't Wait for Health Reform, http://www.catholichealthcare.us/. Accessed December 17, 2009.

43. Laurie Goodstein, "U.S. Nuns Facing Vatican Scrutiny," *New York Times*, July 2, 2009; Thomas C. Fox, "Women Religious Not Complying with Vatican Study," *National Catholic Reporter*, n.d., http://ncronline.org/pring/15950. Accessed December 18, 2009; Patricia Montemurri, "Progressive Adrian Nuns under Vatican Scrutiny," *Detroit Free Press*, May 24, 2010.

Index

Note: A *t* after a page number denotes a table on that page.

About the Author

Barbra Mann Wall, PhD, RN, FAAN, is an associate professor of nursing and the associate director of the Barbara Bates Center for the Study of the History of Nursing at the University of Pennsylvania. She received her BS in nursing from the University of Texas at Austin, her MS in nursing from Texas Woman's University, and her PhD in history from the University of Notre Dame. Her extensive body of work, which includes award-winning books, manuscripts, and presentations around the globe, has helped stimulate debates on the health care policy of many countries pertinent to the role and interactions of government with religious and secular enterprises.

Available titles in the Critical Issues in Health and Medicine series:

David Mechanic, *The Truth about Health Care: Why Reform Is Not Working in America*

Alyssa Picard, *Making the American Mouth: Dentists and Public Health in the Twentieth Century*

David J. Rothman and David Blumenthal, *Medical Professionalism in the New Information Age*

Karen Seccombe and Kim A. Hoffman, *Just Don't Get Sick: Access to Health Care in the Aftermath of Welfare Reform*

Leo B. Slater, *War and Disease: Biomedical Research on Malaria in the Twentieth Century*

Rosemary A. Stevens, Charles E. Rosenberg, and Lawton R. Burns, eds., *History and Health Policy in the United States: Putting the Past Back In*

Barbra Mann Wall, *American Catholic Hospitals: A Century of Changing Markets and Missions*

CPSIA information can be obtained
at www.ICGtesting.com
Printed in the USA
LVHW030949071218
599532LV00002B/7/P